101 Ways to Find Six-Figure Medical or Popular Ghostwriting Jobs & Clients

101 Ways to Find Six-Figure Medical or Popular Ghostwriting Jobs & Clients

◆

A Step-by-Step Guide

Anne Hart

ASJA Press
New York Lincoln Shanghai

101 Ways to Find Six-Figure Medical or Popular Ghostwriting Jobs & Clients
A Step-by-Step Guide

Copyright © 2006 by Anne Hart

ASJA Press
an imprint of iUniverse, Inc.

iUniverse books may be ordered through booksellers or by contacting:

iUniverse
2021 Pine Lake Road, Suite 100
Lincoln, NE 68512
www.iuniverse.com
1-800-Authors (1-800-288-4677)

ISBN-13: 978-0-595-41679-0
ISBN-10: 0-595-41679-9

Printed in the United States of America

Contents

Medical Ghostwriting

How would you like to write regulatory copy and earn perhaps $100,000 annually as a medical ghostwriter? You'd be writing anything from pharmaceutical reports to informational books by scientists, physicians, and researchers. You could work with pharmaceutical firms, medical software manufacturers, or for public relations firms or literary agents. You'd be making a lot more than the usual $10,000 a ghostwriter may receive for writing a career development how-to book. Medical ghostwriters can receive up to $20,000 per report. You'll be writing research reports in a formal style.

Those reports will be sent to a variety of regulatory agencies. The purpose of the report is to allow regulators to review new pharmaceutical products or medical gadgets before they reach consumers. See the article titled, *C. P. Scope And Impact Of Financial Conflicts Of Interest In Biomedical Research* by Bekelman, J.E., Li, Y. and Gross, Journal of the American Medical Association 289: 454-465.

You'll be analyzing a lot of project data looking for results from a variety of clinical trials. Physicians and statisticians would be interviewed. In addition to ghostwriting results of clinical trials reports and medical journal articles, you'll work creatively to produce print ads for pharmaceutical firms. Like a journalist, you'll be writing and editing articles to be reviewed by medical peer review journals, and you'll write the 'copy' for displays set up as exhibits at medical conventions. These are called poster sessions. The convention center's halls are bedecked with posters explaining outcomes of clinical research trials and other projects.

You know you have the aptitude to become a medical writer or medical ghostwriter if paying attention to scientific detail and analyzing numbers and words and then writing about it with clarity are your best abilities. It's similar to being a technical writer, but emphasizes writing about medicine—the results of medical trials—instead of writing computer or engineering manuals. You'll need to understand and analyze the data.

For more information on what preparation you'll need, you can contact the American Medical Writers Association and take as many seminars at what's offered during conferences or other courses in your university on the subject of regulatory medical writing. Seek out internships doing or working with medical writing at various clinical services departments within some of the larger pharmaceutical firms. See the article written by D. Willman titled, *Stealth Merger: Drug Companies and Government Medical Research.* Los Angeles Times. 2003 Dec 7: A1, A32-3.

You can also work in the nutraceutical industry or in the vaccine rather than the drug manufacturing division of the pharmaceutical industry. Working with the pharmaceutical giants is where the higher pay is. In contrast, working with a small firm or with the government regulatory agencies may have varying results as far as your income.

Currently, trained, experienced medical ghostwriters are in demand. For bench scientists who have had problems finding the type of job they want, medical writing is one alternative career track. For journalists unhappy with the downsizing and merging of general newspapers and magazines, going back to school to take courses in one of the life sciences or pharmacy is another possibility.

For registered nurses with master's degrees, medical writing is an alternative career. There are nurses who entered the field of medical ghostwriting by recruiting potential patients for clinical trials and decided to study more life science and medical writing and focus on finding a way to get an assignment and the proper training to write medical regulatory reports. There are alternative ways of entering the field as long as you can analyze and understand the data or find a way to learn the skills you must do well on the job under the tight time pressure and long hours.

Currently most medical writers earning six-figure incomes are writing regulatory copy. Most of those who write regulatory copy have at least a master's degree. Medical ghostwriters most likely have majored in any of the life sciences such as biology or genetics. Almost a third of those writing regulatory copy have a PhD in pharmacy.

So if all you have is a master's in English with emphasis on professional or creative writing or a journalism degree, you'll have to take courses in a life science to even the playing field with those who have a master's degree in a life science and perhaps a minor in medical writing.

Some of the newer master's degree programs in medical writing do let you combine life science courses with writing courses. Another way to get your foot in the door is to audit courses in the life sciences. That way, you can get in the field as a writer using your writing degree and focus on learning to meticulously interpret numerical data along with the scientific and medical terminology familiar to life science majors.

There is an open door in the field, but you will be competing with trained scientists who enjoy ghostwriting. There are several different ways to read enough science textbooks to understand the regulatory reports. You can start by reading these types of reports and finding out how to interpret the numerical data and medical terminology. Start by reading formal reports submitted to a variety of regulatory agencies. One example is to read what is submitted to the Food and Drug Administration (FDA).

Learn how the FDA reviews new products. When they analyze the report, for what are they looking? Look at sample reports and find out what courses you need to take to catch up in your ability to review and write about new products and devices. You might want to find out how regulators analyze what medical ghostwriters have written.

Break down each step of the report. You know that it is an analysis. You know it is supposed to interpret data results from clinical trials. Talk to or interview people who work with clinical trials. Volunteer to work with them on various committees or associations and look at what is ghostwritten in those clinical trials results. Talk to the physicians who work on the projects and take a course in interpreting statistics. Talk to the statisticians who work on these projects.

Unless you're an intern working for college credit, most will be too busy to give you an informational interview. So approach them as a networking situation at a professional association member. Join associations for medical writers or do freelance writing for newsletters or other publications that allow you to attend medical conferences and cover what is presented. You can talk to these people at conventions when they are not under tight time pressure at work.

One of the reasons that medical ghostwriters are paid six figures is that they are under time pressures. Pharmaceutical medical writers and ghostwriters earn from $75,000 to $120,000 annually once they are experienced and in a stable job. Medical writing managers are the ones earning the $120,000 range incomes, not the beginners. If the time pressure is too stressful, you can always go into medical sales and travel the world.

Medical writing (or ghostwriting) is one career alternative for bench scientists who would rather write than work on laboratory experiments. It's also an alternative for physicians. And for journalists who can take a double major in journalism and a life science, such as biology or organic chemistry or earn a master's degree in medical writing, it's a career track with an open door. If you want to work with medical books and don't have any science courses, but really love to read about science, consider becoming a medical book indexer.

If you have a science background and would rather edit than write, consider becoming a medical textbook editor. For those on their way up in a career track, starting as a medical proofreader or editorial assistant is one foot in the door to a medical ghostwriting career track.

There Are Two Types of Medical Writing

Choose whether you want to do scientific medical writing or marketing medical writing. The American Medical Writers Association explains the difference between scientific medical writing and marketing medical writing on its Web site at: http://www.amwa-dvc.org/toolkit/index.shtml. Just click on the link at the Web site of the American Medical Writers Association and read about the various types of medical writing career track choices. It's self-explanatory.

Scientific medical writers work with analytical and numerical data. Marketing medical writers focus on developing and publishing promotional, marketing, advertising, public relations, media news releases, and sales data. Scientific Medical writing and ghostwriting does include writing advertising copy for pharmaceuticals and medical devices.

Scientific medical writing requires a good knowledge of science since you'll be writing the scientific or medical language content for DVDs and CDs as well as Web content. You'll be writing medical journal articles, usually as a ghostwriter. Your job may entail a lot of editing, writing abstracts for medical journals, and medical education materials read by physicians, nurses, and scientists.

You may also write patient education materials. That's why registered nurses who are used to writing patient educational materials and various therapists in patient education may find a career in writing patient education training publications.

Writing Monographs

You'll write monographs, usually on one subject that might be used to inform and educate physicians, nurses, health care workers, regulatory agencies, and patients. According to the free Wikipedia encyclopedia online at: http://en.wikipedia.org/wiki/Monograph: "A monograph is a scholarly book or a treatise on a single subject, class of subjects, or person." It is a one-time publication that is complete in itself. A more specific definition is: "a lengthy work on a particular subject or person, detailed in treatment and often containing bibliographies."

In addition to monographs, you'll be writing medical educational materials that will be put on DVDs and CDs. You'll write content for the Web, abstracts for medical journals, medical journal articles—ghostwritten,

What Materials Will You Develop?

You'll be writing and designing multimedia materials, pharmaceutical advertising and marketing, speeches for physicians that you'll ghostwrite. The physician, not you will get the credit for the speech and any medical journal articles or abstracts you will write. You'll write scripts and presentations for multimedia projects, marketing and advertising copy for pharmaceutical projects, material for posters, regulatory documents; clinical trial reports, integrated summaries of safety, efficacy, investigator brochures and documents for investigational new drugs, new drug application submissions, and protocols. Additionally, you'll be writing the copy that goes on slide kits and selecting or arranging the slides or other graphics. You'll write and organize sales training manuals and white papers. All this will be done under the pressure of time. And you'll work long hours to meet the schedule.

Employers

You'll apply for ghostwriting jobs at the larger pharmaceutical firms, hospitals, health care systems, medical public relations and advertising agencies, medical education publishers and distributors, contract research organizations, professional associations, teaching hospitals and academic medical centers, health foundations, and managed care corporations. Other ghostwriting jobs are found at more generalized publishers. Content producers are hired by Web site hosting firms that are under contract with medical and pharmaceutical corporations. You may do editing for a biotech corporation.

Mostly, you'll be re-writing scientific papers, grant proposals, and training a staff in scientific writing or editing. You also can work as a freelance bio-sciences editor, or index medical text books. Ghostwriters also write peer-reviewed manuscripts. You can find work at academic medical centers in the publications department. Some of the highest paying ghostwriting jobs are for the larger pharmaceutical firms and consist of writing pharmaceutical promotional materials, reports, or medical journal articles.

Ghostwriting Jobs in Medical Marketing

Advertising copy, newsletters, patient education publications, public relations releases, proposal writing, proofreading, and training manual writing and editing makes up what medical marketing writers do. A lot of the material will be put on computer discs. You'll also write articles for various types of magazines and marketing publications and prepare training materials.

Medical marketing communicators are hired by various foundations, non-profit agencies, medical advertising and public relations agencies, and some pharmaceutical firms. Mostly it will be publishers for whom you'll write. There will be Web site content to produce, and some hospitals and health care corporations hire medical marketing writers for their public relations departments. Academic medical centers and teaching hospitals also need editors and proofreaders, book indexers, and other communicators. Managed care organizations hire writers for their marketing communications departments as do medical software manufacturers.

Medical marketing doesn't require as in-depth science training as scientific medical writing employers may require. Nurses and respiratory therapists or other types of therapists with a writing background sometimes enter medical marketing to write patient education materials. For example, a respiratory therapist or registered nurse with teaching experience or registered dietician may finish a master's degree in medical writing and find work writing consumer education material for publishers or Web sites. Medical marketing writers often write press releases and make press kits for academic medical centers or teaching hospitals and nonprofit agencies.

Articles written for general consumer magazines and newspapers are written by journalists who have entered the field of medical marketing writing by writing for medical newspapers. Often they are sent to cover medical conventions for a periodical.

There are some jobs for medical marketing writers with pharmaceutical firms and healthcare programs in their education, training, or public relations department focusing on medical communications. Ghostwriters and freelancers may write for medical book publishers or write for consumer magazines or contribute to multi-authored books. The American Medical Writer's Association has a job-related division that you may want to explore to find out what various types of employment is open to medical marketing communicators.

What will you write as a medical ghostwriter?

Abstracts

Advertising copy

Books and Book Chapters

Brochures

Clinical Trial Copy, Ads, and Reports

Editorial Position Statements

FAQs

Grants

Journal Articles

Manuals

Meeting Summaries

Monographs

Newsletters

Patient Education Material

Pharmaceutical Clinical Trial Reports

Podcasts

Posters

Product Information

Regulatory Peer Review Reports

Reports

Scripts

Slide Kits

Statistical Reports

Transcripts

Websites

White Papers

◆   ◆   ◆

You'll never see your name/byline on a pharmaceutical report because the physicians for whom you ghostwrote the report will receive recognition from being published under their own names. In a "publish or perish" world of science and academia, research and manufacturing, ghostwriting medical information is big business.

It's a way that pharmaceutical manufacturers can communicate with physicians. If you want to ghostwrite in this field, you'll have to investigate for yourself the process of what information physicians receive and who wrote it.

To earn this type of money, frequently, you'd be hired if you had a master's degree or PhD in one of the life sciences with a minor in medical, science, or technical writing (or several courses in journalism). Some universities offer undergraduate degrees in medical writing where you can combine writing and editing courses with life science courses in a double major.

Continuing education courses and seminars are offered by national associations such as the American Medical Writers Association. Whether you'd be hired and where you'll be working—in what department of a pharmaceutical company depends upon what type of writing you'll be doing.

Also see the professional science master's degree program discussed at the Professional Master's Web site at: http://www.sciencemasters.com/. The New York-based Alfred P. Sloan Foundation has helped launch new M.S. degrees in 45 institutions with strong graduate programs in the sciences and mathematics. With a minor in medical writing or journalism, you have excellent preparation for a career as a medical ghostwriter. The CNN Money.com Web site at: http://money.cnn.com/2004/09/08/pf/sixfigs_seven/index.htm discusses six-figure medical writers in the pharmaceutical industry.

You can even earn graduate degrees in medical or science writing and ask for an internship with a large pharmaceutical firm where you may ask to work in the department that develops the pharmaceutical reports given to physicians and pharmacists.

With few or no science courses, medical writers usually are put in the public relations department of a pharmaceutical firm. Each company has its own specifications of what it takes to ghostwrite medical reports. Do you always have to have a PhD? No. But you do need to understand the scientific material and write clearly to communicate with physicians.

The best way to find out is to call the pharmaceutical firm for whom you want to work and ask whether someone with your background and education or experience would be hired to ghostwrite medical reports or other materials and how much would you be paid compared to someone with a graduate degree in the life sciences.

You can compare the work of ghostwriters with a science degree or experience to the work of ghostwriters with a degree in English or medical writing. You could ask human resource departments of the larger pharmaceutical firms whether there's a difference in pay between someone with an undergraduate degree compared to someone with a masters degree.

Numerous medical report ghostwriters have masters' degrees in a science such as chemistry and are familiar with pharmaceutical research, design, and synthesis. Because of good writing skills, they may be hired as ghostwriters. Other ghostwriters come from a background with an interest in science and understanding of it, but actual coursework in writing.

Another open door is in medical indexing and editing of textbooks. However, the big and steady money is in medical ghostwriting of pharmaceutical reports for physicians.

You won't be getting your byline in print or royalties, but if you specialize in medical ghostwriting, you have a one-upmanship leg over the ghost writer who writes memoirs of celebrities for high fees, because there is a lot less competition for medical ghostwriting than there is to compete with established celebrity biographers in Hollywood and New York to write news stories, true crime, or memoirs of celebrities and other famous personalities or politicians in the current media spotlight.

Pharmaceutical companies hire ghostwriters to write reports and articles. Many drug review articles are written by ghostwriters. See The Guardian Unlimited Web site at: http://observer.guardian.co.uk/uk_news/story/0,6903,1101680,00.html and read the article from the Observer titled, *"Revealed: how drug firms 'hoodwink' medical journals: Pharmaceutical giants hire ghostwriters to produce articles—then put doctors' names on them,"* by Antony Barnett, public affairs editor, Sunday December 7, 2003.

The article reports that "estimates suggest" that "nearly 50 percent" of all articles published in medical journals are by penned ghostwriters, not written by physicians or scientific researchers that also are academics.

The question now for future medical ghostwriters is to find out what type of education and experience are the "pharmaceutical giants" looking for when they hire ghostwriters to write medical journal articles or other pharmaceutical reports that are intended for an audience of physicians and scientists?

If you read an article by a physician with an MD after his or her name or a PhD, do you wonder whether the ghostwriter hired to write the journal article has the same training or needs the same training to verify the facts in the article—the positive and negative—as the physician or scientist whose name and byline appears on the journal article?

And if you're planning to become a medical ghostwriter, how do you prepare for this type of work? You don't need to go to medical school, but there are physicians who would rather write than practice medicine who do ghostwriting. Other ghostwriters have undergraduate or graduate degrees in one of the sciences, and not necessarily a PhD.

What does it take to become a medical ghostwriter and be hired by the largest pharmaceutical firms that pay comfortable incomes and offer steady employment to ghostwriters? It sure beats competing with the Hollywood crowd to get assignments from publishers to ghostwrite novels for celebrities, or does it, in terms of steady work and relatively long-term income?

If you like to keep learning current scientific information as you write, consider a career as a medical ghostwriter. See the article by Antony Barnett titled, *Revealed: How Drug Firms 'Hoodwink' Medical Journals. Pharmaceutical giants hire ghostwriters to produce articles—then put doctors' names on them.* The Observer. Sunday December 7, 2003.

◆   ◆   ◆

Twenty-Four Topics Beginning Ghostwriters Want to Discuss with Experts

1.   How Much to Charge for Ghostwriting

2.   Where to Find Popular Clients or Publishers & Who Are Their Audiences?

3.   How to Get an Assignment

4.   How to Hone Training and Specialize

5.   Ghostwriting Books, Proposals & Query Letters

6.   Ghostwriting Speeches

7.   Ghostwriting Booklets or Brochures

8.   Ghost Copywriting

9.   Ghostwriting Newsletters

10. Coaching For Key Topics

◆   ◆   ◆

Replies to the 24 Discussion Topics

1. How Much to Charge for Ghostwriting

For non-medical ghostwriting, charge one to three dollars a word or a flat fee of $10,000 and up. If a publisher normally gives an author a $5,000 advance and 5% to 12% royalties, a ghostwriter who will not receive recognition, byline, or royalties needs to ask for a flat fee to compensate, starting at double the advance of the author in average advances. Most writers are offered for how-to books $3,000 to $7,500 in advance.

They will get royalties, but the royalties may also be only 12% and 15% of advance and royalty amounts may have to be paid to the literary agent if there is an agent. There may be co-authors on a project that split everything 50-50.

If you are the only ghostwriter on the project, ask for double the advance as a flat fee or a per word basis. Usually $2 a word may be settled upon for a book, or a flat fee of $10,000 or more.

Figure a 70,000 word book at $2 a word would amount to $140,000. No publisher will pay that on a how-to book that may bring in only $240 per year in royalties for the author.

Instead, you'll be paid a flat fee of perhaps $10,000 which would be double the average $5,000 advance for a trade paperback how-to book. Work out the flat fee with the publisher. This usually would be twice what the author would get if the book was not ghostwritten and the author was going to receive royalties.

Flat fees are given on books, and dollars per word are given on shorter projects such as brochures, greeting cards, or even 15-page booklets. Each publisher and agent would be different and negotiate a different price to pay you as a ghostwriter. If you join organizations of ghostwriters, you can discuss what most of them are getting for similar types of projects.

For information on medical editing, check out the Council of Biology Editors at: http://www.monroecc.edu/depts/library/cbe.htm.

For Medical Ghostwriting

You earn the most money on a steady basis by ghostwriting medical reports. Freelancers might charge a familiar $35 per hour. However, book projects come and go. Report ghostwriting is steadier by comparison.

Epigenetics is a new field for medical ghostwriters to cover, particularly any area of research related to the study of the epigenome. Epigenetics and epigenomics include studies of changes in gene silencing. That term 'silencing' refers to the chemicals that switch genes on or off.

Sometimes the genes switch on or off when certain nutrients, supplements, or special prenatal diets are given to expectant mothers. Animals are tested first in epigenetic research. The turning on or off of genes or 'silencing' usually occurs without changes in the genes themselves.

Epigenetics is a new field ripe for medical ghostwriters, considering all the therapies and studies focused on switching these genes back on or off. Medical ghostwriters might emphasize how epigenetics or other studies of the epigenome could be used to treat aging, inherited diseases and cancer.

See the article titled *"Inside the Business of Medical Ghostwriting"* by reporter: Erica Johnson; Producer: Michael Gruzuk; Researcher: Colman Jones, on the CBC Marketplace: Health: Medical Ghostwriting at the Web site at: http://www.cbc.ca/consumers/market/files/health/ghostwriting/. It's true that medical ghostwriters can earn $100,000 annually writing reports for some of the large pharmaceutical companies. But you'd need an hourly or flat-fee contract for out-sourcing, freelance work, or permanent employment.

You won't earn royalties from medical ghostwriting. If you request royalties, you would also request your own byline or byline with a co-author. You'd need a contract, and copyright, preferably in your name and the co-author's on a per-centage basis, usually 50-50.

Most medical ghostwriters work on a flat-fee basis or a special arrangement with a pharmaceutical firm. Most medical ghostwriters don't earn royalties.

Pharmaceutical manufacturers frequently employ medical ghostwriters as per-manent staff. Your credibility as a medical ghostwriter depends upon how much you can be trusted to know and check your facts, your scientific protocols, and the credibility of those supplying your 'unflawed' research materials and results of studies.

You can read the article on what type of reports a ghostwriter is expected to write. The best way to prepare for a career as a medical ghostwriting is to com-bine writing courses with life science courses. Managers can earn up to $120,000 annually. It depends upon the company.

If you can attend a college of pharmacy or major in chemistry or other life sci-ences (biology or genetics) and minor in journalism, medical writing, or technical writing, work on the newsletters published by professional associations and intern in medical writing with a pharmaceutical company, you have an excellent route in. Of course, there are PhDs in life sciences, physicians, nurses, and pharmacists in the field competing with people who have an undergraduate degree in medical writing.

Most medical writers with a degree in English or medical writing or technical writing and few or no science courses are placed in the public relations depart-ment of the larger pharmaceutical companies. You can get a foot in the door, but it's usually by applying for a job ghostwriting reports for pharmaceutical firms, especially the larger ones. See the article by Shannon Brownlee titled, *Doctors Without Borders. Why You Can't Trust Medical Journals Anymore*. Washington Monthly. April 2003.

How Much to Charge for General Ghostwriting

The two biggest problems ghostwriters contend with is paring down redundancy—repetition in a speech, book, or article and inconsistencies in memoirs and novels and listening with an 'ear' for how the ghostwritten work portrays the 'voice' of resilience (point of view and style) of the non-silent author. You're hired to write and eliminate redundancy.

You also must play editor and organize similar topics that have to be grouped together. You must check for indents and other spacing problems such as too many "hard returns" on the keyboard, tab spacing, spelling errors, word usage, and grammar inconsistencies in the notes or recorded voice of a professional or entrepreneur. Other times a ghostwriter is hired to write an entire book, booklet, speech, or article from scratch based on recorded interviews.

You're paid to be highly creative and down-to-earth factual, stable and under control. Your writing must be animated, not flat, and you have to satisfy your client's wishes as to how the book sounds to the outside world. You must follow directions and yet be visionary, be charismatic in print, and promote what your client is offering with facts that can be checked for credibility. You represent your client's reputation and career.

The client, also called the primary author most likely has an agent and a publisher, but needs a silent co-author—a ghostwriter—whose name will never appear on the book to partner on a book-to-book or project-to-project basis. A literary agent or a celebrity's manager may be the person most likely to ask you to ghostwrite a book. Sometimes, a physician, nutritionist, traveler, executive, entrepreneur, video producer, or any type of scientist may seek out a medical ghostwriter. You may be contacted by someone who has been in the news, or a politician. Usually, though, you'll have to let others know you're a ghostwriter because you'll be invisible.

Begin Ghostwriting By Contacting Owners of Public Relations Agencies with Celebrity Clients

To become a general ghostwriter, not necessary a medical ghostwriter, start by contacting public relations agency owners who deal mostly with celebrities. They often have requests to write how-to books by the celebrities they represent.

With experience, you can move on to writing the memoirs of entertainers or other celebrities in the news. Public relations agencies that publish books with information about celebrities are a good start for beginning ghostwriters trying to break in. The first book assignments you get may be writing how-to books on careers for celebrity clients or other publicists working for a larger agency. The next hurdle is writing the memoirs of celebrities.

Ghostwriters may be chosen from a team or pool of writers who specialize in biographies of entertainers or other figures in the news. You may be hired to write speeches, books, booklets, articles, annual business reports, scripts, multimedia presentations, learning materials, news releases, and more for professionals, publishers, and corporate executives.

What might you expect to hear as a ghostwriter from the author with whom you are partnered for a project? There are lots of humorous situations you'll find when ghostwriting.

Below is an example of a humorous conversational example sent to me as email from one ghostwriter who has asked to be listed as anonymous.

Hi Anne!

A few horror stories…

Me: So in the proposal, you have a chapter called Creative Resilience. Could you tell me something about that?

Expert: Well, when we need to be resilient, it's important to get creative.
(long pause…)

Me: Do you have anything to add to that?
Expert: Um, not really.

Me: Sooo…this would be more of a sentence than a chapter?
Expert: Yeah, I think so.

Another funny one:

The expert who had her elderly father who she said was "really smart" faxed me his scribbled and cryptic notes on the meaning of life, and asked me if that could be "worked into the book somewhere." When I asked her to give me her thoughts on what he had written (as I couldn't make heads or tails out of it), she had none.

    Same expert asked one of her friends to write a "corrected" version of a Buddhist-type teaching story I had put in her book at her bequest. You see, the friend knew I got it "wrong" because she'd seen it on CSI or some show like that a few weeks before. (I found 4 versions on the Internet)

    Same expert had to write a chapter on a particular subject and asked me to go to the bookstore and see what other people had written so she could get some ideas on what she wanted to say in her book of advice to the masses.

Q. Most ghostwriters are invisible. Here's the chance to write about what you enjoy most about ghostwriting. What's the most important lesson you've learned from life as a ghostwriter?

1. *Don't get involved if there is no time to write it and way too much money involved, even if your cut of the advance is a big one. The pressure of time and a*

*ridiculously large advance will fall on YOU, unfair though it may be. You'll be
expected to work miracles overnight.*

2. *If you can't get the expert to give you SPECIFIC ideas that would work as bullet
    points under each of his chapter ideas in the proposal, it doesn't matter if everyone
    is over the moon about the proposal. YOU judge the proposal, and YOU find out
    what the expert's main ideas are. If they're awfully fuzzy, listen to your instincts
    and say "no."*

3. *Do not do a minute's worth of work until the check to you has cleared. Period.
    No excuses. It's not your problem that the author's contract with the publisher has
    been held up, or that the agency can't front you the money for your first payment,
    and that the author is sooooo strapped for money this month. Let them find some-
    one else to do it, if they can't pay you from the moment you begin work, forget
    them.*

4. *Be very careful about plagiarism. Experts who are not writers are prone to acci-
    dentally plagiarizing from the Internet or from other authors. If it doesn't sound
    like they wrote it, they probably didn't.*

5. *When the agent and editor say they want you to capture the expert's "voice," they
    don't mean his actual voice, they mean the voice he would ideally have given
    what their flap copy has to say about him. Throw in his catchphrases to make it
    sound like "him," but the actual voice should not sound like how he actually talks
    or, god forbid, writes.*

6. *Ask the expert why he wants a ghostwriter. If it's being imposed upon him by the
    publisher and you sense he has airs about being an author, RUN.*

Q. How Much Do You Charge?

*Usually, it's a flat fee. Sometimes, I've done deals where the flat fee is based on a cer-
tain number of my hours at my hourly rate, and the author and I work together to
estimate the time needed and we communicate when I'm running short or long, and
in the end, they pay me according to my actual hours. If I'm short, they may "bank"
their hours for use on the next project (this is only for clients who write multiple books
with me).*

*I have not yet written speeches or booklets or brochures. Once, I did ghost an article
for a book I'd edited. I've never worked with a PR agency. I've ghosted books by professionals and a semi-celebrity.*

◆   ◆   ◆

Ghostwriters as Surrogate Parents

Here's an e-letter from a ghostwriter on a variety of subjects who has given permission for her name and business location to be mentioned in this book:

Hello Anne

The aspect of ghostwriting that I enjoy the most is being a surrogate mother for someone else's literary baby. While their ideas are wonderful, my clients lack the ability to conceive a book project from start to finish and to write with polish and panache. As a ghost, I transform a client's scribbled notes into a fully developed book manuscript; in doing so, I bring a client's ideas to life on the printed page.

Pauline Bartel, M.A.
Bartel Communications, Inc.
12-1/2 Division Street
Waterford, NY 12188
www.paulinebartel.com

Certified by Albany County and New York State
as a Woman-Owned Business Enterprise (WBE)

Winner of Awards of Distinction from The Communicator Awards 2006 Print Competition

◆   ◆   ◆

How Much to Charge Depends upon What Your Client Will Pay for Visibility

You have the choice to charge by a day rate or by the word. Corporate ghostwriting usually offers you a flat fee or hourly amount. If your manuscript goes through several iterations (revisions) before approved by a group, a corporation, or even one person, you'll get more money charging an hourly amount. Be sure to specify in your contract that you'll be paid an hourly amount for each revision of your manuscript.

Ghostwriters are outsiders brought into a corporation or nonprofit agency to present favorable images and words. You are either looked upon by a company as an outsider who might make more trouble than you are worth because you haven't been an insider long enough.

Or you're looked upon as a connecting bridge. The bridge is there to convince, promote, and represent the company's image, reliability, and credibility to the world. You're there to connect the outside world to what benefits the company offers. Using words and images, you share meaning. You communicate. And you are paid according to the results the company gets from your words.

◆   ◆   ◆

Rates: Ghostwriting White Papers and Annual Reports

In a corporate setting you'll be ghostwriting annual reports and "white papers" for an executive, committee, or group. You'll also be ghostwriting articles and perhaps speeches, presentations, or scripts for slide shows and training videos. Articles and white papers usually offer you pay based on a per-word basis.

When ghostwriting sales letters, charge by the hour. Direct mail marketing and other types of sales letters may be ghostwritten for advertising agencies and marketing firms. In an advertising agency or marketing corporation, you probably will be paid by the day for ghostwriting. If you're experienced, the current rate is about $500 to $600 per day. At this high-end rate, you'll be coming into an office and working under supervision so your hours can be clocked. See Shane Ellison's Web site, *How Drug Companies Deceive Doctors, Revised Edition, 2005* at: http://www.newswithviews.com/Ellison/shane20.htm#_ftn4.

Rates: Ghostwriting Speeches

Doing corporate work requires negotiation on contracts. If you know more about the business or product that the managers, you can negotiate on a per-day fee basis. Corporate ghostwriting often requires speech writing. The current rate for experienced corporate speechwriters is about $1,000 per day to write a five-minute speech.

At the $1,000 per day rate, make sure there is no fluff, unnecessary, or distracting words in your speech. A five-minute speech must pack in the most important points the corporation wants to make about a product, service, or situation.

How to Evaluate Your Ghostwritten Speech

Read your speech aloud and record it. Play it back and listen how it sounds to the ear. Ask several listeners to give you feedback before you cut and revise. What you're looking for is not only effective words but the cadence and rhythm of the speech. Listen to what you write by reading it aloud and playing it back several times. Is it smooth and consistent?

Your goal is efficacy. Pare the words to bare bones. Look for impact. Keep sentences short and simple. Use two-sentence paragraphs. Here are 20 pointers to consider before ghostwriting speeches.

What Angles Will You Use on Each Speech, Book, Booklet, Brochure, or Feature Article Paragraph?

1. Look for the angles or slant on each speech paragraph. To listen for the first impression or impact, set up your audio recorder and read your speech directly into the microphone. Listen for ease of understanding.

2. Without being simplistic, you need to use plain language and simple concepts that are easy to understand at first listening. Your goal is to be understood immediately without having to explain or repeat information. The less complex your speech, the more people will look at how practical are the solutions you're offering.

3. Use only necessary words, and define any words that the average person may not understand immediately. Keep stress levels low for listeners. Copywriting techniques work well in speech writing.

4. Communicate succinctly by inspiring creative, yet practical applications of ideas by your audience.

5. Understand why people would be interested in hearing the speech.

6. Identify all the key messages and put them in your first paragraph.

7. Every audience has its own style. Every client or corporation has its own style. Find that style and write in a way that fits in with the group.

8. Don't overwhelm the audience with technology applications, unless your audience is made up of technical-oriented people.

9. Use specific angles in each opening and new paragraph. You can find out which angles to use by making a list of the interests of the listeners. Match the speaker to the audience before you write.

10. Find out who will be invited and how their interests or occupations fit into your speech.

11. Select the correct tone for your audience. Every speech has its own tone. Who will be listening and what are their interests?

12. Use brainstorming techniques with your client before writing a speech.

13. Write persuasively. What coaching has your client had?

14. Match the speech with the client's character. Use the speech manuscript in a newsletter.

15. Write the beginning paragraphs of the speech using headlines. For example, if each paragraph is two sentences in length, and each sentence is ten words or less, the first sentence of each paragraph can be a headline that summarizes and emphasizes the message in the paragraph.

16. Offer foresight, insight, and hindsight—pitfalls to avoid.

17. Use picture stories in speech writing to turn pictures back into vivid words that paint pictures. Dress paragraphs in a speech in the same way as a journalist dresses articles.

18. Put the most important information in the first sentence of each paragraph as if it were a headline meant to make an impact on the listener—to bring the audience to attention and focus. Dress your speech before you present it. Clothe your speech in imagery that makes a statement denoting and connoting your message by using concrete, specific details, facts and information that offers direction.

19. Solve problems and show results in a speech. If you find flaws in research, supply believable facts that easily can be checked.

20. Use humor when appropriate. Find a need and supply that need to the audience, which is usually a credible solution to a common problem. Keep your speech light enough to be upbeat, and end with humor, if inappropriate to the occasion, use uplifting, specific examples for the audience to follow or investigate.

21. You're mostly hired in the beginning by public relations firms that have celebrity clients and/or publish directories or books about celebrities.

22. Ghostwriters may open their own public relations agencies.

23. Contact video producers and TV talk shows to work with the media in promoting your client.

24. Accuracy and credibility are your goals. Ghostwriters may stay totally invisible and not promote their clients by remaining in the background. There are two roads to choose. By remaining invisible, you get to write books without being singled out as the author and challenged on the opinions or facts in the book. Make sure what you write can be fact-checked and is credible. Have this put in your contract—that you will not write simply what told to write, but need to be sure the facts can be checked by you for accuracy and proper sources.

Rates: Ghostwriting Corporate Web Pages

When writing corporate Web pages, you become a "content writer" charging by the hour. The current rate is about $100 per hour. Rates vary tremendously with the size of the corporation, the geographic location, and your experience.

If you work an eight-hour day at $100 an hour, billing $800 a day is expected. Let the managers know what you'll bill for an eight-hour day if the project will take you eight hours.

Rates: Word Count

Short word count items such as Web pages, sales letters, news releases, or brief feature articles allow you to invoice your employers by the hour. Most short projects require several revisions and lots of rewriting before they are approved.

To begin, write a series of laminated completed writing samples and put them in a loose leaf binder to show as a portfolio. In your portfolio place sample sales letters, news releases, articles, speeches, Web content, white papers, booklets, brochures, and the first three chapters of a bound paperback book you can photocopy, as well as a sampling of annual reports you've written for a particular industry that you know well.

Estimate Your Hours

Develop templates for time budgets as well as money budgets. Estimate the hours you'll need to complete the project and show the rates for the various hours.

To find out how many hours a project would be required to complete, interview key people for specific information needed in order to research the project. A book would be invoiced by you as a flat fee item. A short content item such as a Web page, sales letter, or five-minute speech, would be billed hourly as your project rate.

You actually do not tell anyone how many hours you think that you'll be working and writing. Don't tell anyone an hourly rate or hours expected to do the job unless you specifically are going to bill your client for hourly work.

Bill at the flat fee rate if you're going to invoice for a book, booklet, script, learning materials, white paper, annual report, or anything not done by hourly. If you don't know how many hours you'll be working, you can't give your client an estimate of how many hours you'll need and how much you'll charge.

For a long-term project such as a book, a flat fee works better. For a five-minute speech, bill at an hourly rate as speeches have more rewrites and revisions than very large projects. A five-minute speech takes hours to write, even before the revisions start. Word choice and emphasis is everything. If humor is added, then the timing plays a part.

If you are writing stand-up comedy material, bill hourly based on revisions that you will be paid for, as long as you include in your contract that you are to be paid for revisions and/or rewrites. Speech writers sometimes also write comedy routines for stand-up comics along with speech for celebrity roasts.

When you draw up your contract, stipulate how many revisions you'll do. If you don't set a limit, you may find yourself doing way too many. If you're paid for each revision, put in writing any limit to the number of revisions you'll do. This helps to put a cap on what your client will have to pay you to complete the project. You might put in writing in your agreement that after the fifth revision with pay, there won't be any more revisions, and the client will have to accept the project as it is at that point.

Your contract should stipulate when the balance due is to be paid. Most publishers pay a writer for a book in thirds—one third after the manuscript is handed in, one third when the revisions are corrected, and one third when everything is completed and the book goes to press or to the final cover design iteration.

If your client wants you to update the book with revisions every two years, have that put in writing in your contract along with how much you'll be paid in flat fees to freshen or revise the book, booklet, or brochure. You need to put in a date when you'll be paid any other balance due.

What clients want is an approved manuscript completed by the client's due date at the price specified in writing in a contract. Use a template to create your contract. There are blank legal contract templates online. Or ask a paralegal or your attorney to draw up a contract. Most often the corporation, publisher, or individual who hires you will draw up the contract if you send a letter specifying what you want in the contract.

Don't leave the contract to an individual client. You have a template ready, a blank contract where you can fill in the specifics for each different project.

Corporate work pays $2 or $3 per word at the current rate, depending upon the complexity of the project. Articles for trade journals usually are paid at the current rate of $2 or $3 a word. To find out the current rate in your area, ask other ghostwriters what they are being paid for corporate articles that end up in trade publications. Some magazines pay $1 a word, and specialty magazines may pay only a few cents per word. Magazines generally don't pay for rewrites and revisions. You're offered a flat fee.

If you are ghostwriting an article for a client, and the article will end up as a feature article in a trade journal or general popular consumer magazine, you charge your client one fee for writing and revising the article. The magazine that pays only a few cents a word or more will directly pay the author—your client, not you. If the magazine pays very little, but you are paid a lot more for writing the feature article, generally it means that your client wants the publicity for some service, publication, or product in the magazine as promotion.

If you're lucky, the client will ask you to ghostwrite more material and there will be fewer re-writes. If you have been doing technical writing, it gives you practice in what is entailed with ghostwriting. Make sure you list your priorities.

Ghostwriting is about books, articles, or speeches. Corporate ghostwriting is more about annual reports, white papers, and marketing reports. It may also entail writing scripts for corporate training or multimedia for presentations at trade shows and conferences.

Rates for Ghostwriting Annual Reports

One of the highest paying markets for ghostwriting is writing the annual report and billing your client for $4 or more per hour, plus the same for revisions. Another market for ghostwriting is writing direct mail sales letters at similar rates as well as copywriting for other writers—ghost copywriting at $35 and up per hour.

A notoriously lower-paying market is writing trade articles for industrial journals and other trade publications. Annual reports pay highly because you have to hang around a corporation long enough to learn and research detailed regulatory information. You are controlled by constant changing regulatory requirements and can't overlook an important detail that could derail your ghostwriting career early on.

Watch out for blind spots—important information in the regulatory material when you write an annual report. Look at SEC publications to get an idea of how regulatory material is worded. Writing annual reports also is a good field for a writer with training in reading and interpreting the language of regulatory information used by a particular corporation.

You can intern with a company to learn about it or work on the company's newsletter, interview people, and talk with the corporation's attorneys. To start, focus on the nonprofit groups. They can use volunteers, speech writers, or technical editors who want to learn the ropes about the organization. Emphasize writing grant proposals for them.

Take a course in grant proposal writing or read a book on how to write annual reports and grant proposals before you ask to ghostwrite grant proposals for a nonprofit organization. Once you have mastered writing grant proposals, you can move on to annual reports for that same corporation.

You're learning these strategies because it's necessary that you know the company in depth and also the regulatory requirements. Look over what the SEC has sent the organization as far as communications and requirements. When you have mastered writing annual reports for the nonprofits, then move to the for-profit corporations.

Learn about the for-profit firms in a similar way—by reading and working with writers who actually write and/or evaluate their annual reports. Instead of volunteering for a for-profit company as you might with a nonprofit firm, you might work with their public relations department, technical writing division, or marketing arena. Interview or work with their speech writers.

If the speech writer has no time to talk to you, join an association of speech writers and network with speechwriters. Also talk to a company's event planners and paralegal departments, and most relevant of all, watch the corporation's own technical editors write annual reports.

Ghostwriting Booklets and Brochures

Charge your client by the word. The current rate varies from one to three dollars per word. If you are writing only a few words, you may get that rate. But if you're writing many words, per-word rates for booklets generally will vary with what the company is willing to pay based on the corporation's budget for ghostwriting a booklet or brochure. A brochure contains fewer words than a booklet. Most booklets run from 3,000 to 4,000 words, with the average word length at about 3,750-4,000 words.

Page length for booklets average about 15 pages. However, the size of the booklet varies widely. Some booklets are 5 ½ inches by 8 inches. Others are 6 inches by nine inches. Some are narrow and long, and others are wide and short. Brochures could be 5 inches wide by 3 inches in length and rolled up to fit inside of a box. Some booklets or brochures can be in multimedia on a disc that is packaged with another product.

Other sizes could fit into a cylindrical mailing tube. Instructional booklets may be ghostwritten or written by technical writers and packaged with a product. On technical writing, often there is no byline, just the name and address of the manufacturer of a product or appliance.

You have round booklets and brochures with computer discs inserted inside a pocket at the back so that the intended audience can view a video or listen to audio. Some round booklets have a wheel inserted that the viewer/reader can turn to look at various product styles, sizes, definitions, or colors. Brochures as well as booklets can take many shapes and sizes, with round brochures being unusually creative because DVDs or CDs can be inserted or wheels can turn to reveal variations on a theme. The aim is not only branding but also to hold the viewer's attention long enough to look at the informational material inside.

Some booklets are learning materials. All show benefits, advantages, and choices. Some booklets and brochures are informational. Others are directional with information keys. Some take the form of videos shown at trade shows and expos as demonstrations. Others are actual 28 ½ minute video infomercials played on DVD players at trade shows to demonstrate how products or services are used, including benefits and advantages.

What Budget Do You Use to Ghostwrite a Booklet?

Most writers want to know what to charge for writing a booklet. Whether you're ghostwriting or writing under your own byline, you have the choice of asking for a flat fee, such as $10,000 for a 15-page booklet or quoting a word basis, such as $2.25 per word. Ask for $10,000 to $12,000 flat fee to ghostwrite a booklet of 15-20 pages. You won't get any royalties. Another person's name will be on the byline. You won't be the co-author, and you won't have a byline that says by XYZ with ABC. A ghostwriter is totally invisible to the public.

You won't be able to tell the public that you wrote that book, booklet, or brochure. Many times no author's name at all appears on a corporate or nonprofit agency's publication such as a brochure, booklet, annual report, or white paper.

The corporate name and logo appears instead. With a complete book, charge by the word, usually $3 per word or a flat fee.

The royalties on the book will go to the person whose name is on the book. You will not get any royalties. Be sure the flat fee is enough to pay for your research expenses, writing, and covers the cost of revisions and re-writing that you'll have to do. A book, like all other written work will have to be approved by the client and/or any group or corporation with which the client is associated who will be approving the book.

If you are writing a memoirs or autobiography for a celebrity, be sure to get paid in advance, usually one third in advance, one third when you finish half the book, and the last third when the book is completed. After you're paid, be sure you have it written in your contract that you'll be paid for revisions and re-writes until the final draft is approved. Otherwise, your client may ask you to keep revising and re-writing with unlimited iterations and revisions at no pay.

It can be exhausting and daunting. Make sure you get paid each time you re-write.

Hollywood script writers that belong to the Writers Guild have contracts that say that each time they re-write a script they will be paid for the re-write. Make sure that you're not treated any less for your labor. Negotiate contracts that have built-in stipulations in writing that say you will be paid each time you revise and re-write the manuscript until it is finally approved and goes to press.

Otherwise, you'll be asked to keep revising and re-writing over and over until a potentially perfectionist client is or is not satisfied and decides whether or not to pay you. That's why it's essential to put into the contract that you'll receive the same fee with each re-write and revision of the original manuscript.

You can ghostwrite any form of writing—books, screenplays, educational scripts, books, booklets, brochures, biographies, and text materials for training. The more words you use, the more you'll earn writing on a per word basis. If you're not writing too many words, a flat-fee basis is better. One example would be if you're writing 50-100 words for a greeting card company. You'd want a flat fee.

In the beginning of your writing career, magazines might offer you 10 cents a word to write an article under your own name. When ghostwriting, another person's byline will appear.

Perhaps you're ghosting for a celebrity, politician, or physician. You can ask for three dollars per word to ghostwrite. But when the individual sends the article with his/her byline to a magazine, that magazine may pay your client only 10 cents a word to publish the article in a magazine.

The reason why someone would pay you three dollars per word to write a 2,000-word magazine article that he or she is only going to get paid 10 cents a word for is to publicize that person's business, service, book, or product. For example, a physician has a new technique, book, or service and wants publicity and visibility from a top-rated magazine or newspaper with a large circulation.

He or she might prefer to pay you as a ghostwriter three dollars a word ($6,000 total plus re-write fee) to produce a 2,000 word article. It's a less expensive alternative to spending $20,000 for a publicist to write an article for a top general interest consumer magazine and make a few phone calls to get the physician on various TV or radio shows or send out press releases that wouldn't duplicate the publicity department of the physician's publisher that sends out similar press releases for free to the media.

On the other hand, re-write fees might be considerably less than three dollars per word for re-writes. It depends on what is agreed upon by both parties when the contract is being written. Your client may agree to pay you only one or two dollars per word to write an article for a magazine. The more experienced you become as a ghostwriter, the more your reputation and credibility will give you the bargaining power to ask for the three dollars an hour. Top celebrities that earn millions each year have budgets that allow the best ghostwriters to command prestigious fees. It's better to start by asking $3 an hour or $6,000 per each 2,000 words written for magazine articles, brochures, or booklets ghostwritten.

What you really are as a ghostwriter is a publicist and promoter for your client, and you're entitled to command the same fees a public relations agency would ask. To find clients, send your own brochures to:

1. entertainment attorneys

2. book publishers, think tanks, trade journal publishers, general magazines

3. real estate firms, concert hall management firms

4. government, movie producers, advertising agencies

5. public relations corporations

6. professional associations for networking

7. marketing firms

8. book packagers and literary agents

9. publicity departments of various industries

10. trade journals

11. physicians associations

12. public speakers' bureaus

13. universities and university presses

14. celebrity managers, celebrity unions and guilds

15. politicians, political parties

16. nonprofit agencies

17. publications, media—TV, radio, and multimedia organizations

18. industry

19. Web sites and Web logs (blogs) seeking content producers or content

20. bookstores, booksellers, distributors university bookstores, and discount or department stores

21. libraries: school, university, and public libraries

22. teachers, professors, trainers, and other educators and educational materials purchasers

23. video producers and distributors, software stores, software manufacturers

24. conference and convention event planners

25. employee newsletter publishers and editors

You may find clients in unusual places such as with organizations for owners of shopping malls, retired professionals associations, scientific groups, tabloid publishers, and academia. What you're looking for are connections.

Musicians, singers, actors, comedians, public speakers, TV clergy, or other celebrities and entertainers and their agents also have clients that might want their life stories published or brochures on their latest album written by ghostwriters.

Some hidden markets include retired celebrities and veterans, physicians and scientists writing about genetics, fertility, or various healing discoveries, such as the latest in botanical herbs and fruit juices, environmentalists, and those involved in alternative healing research that have information they want written by professional ghostwriters.

When you charge a client for ghostwriting a booklet, you can point out that the features to be considered have to be organized on paper according to the topic. For example, if you are ghostwriting a how-to booklet on a product, you have to list the layout plans for the design and for the topic.

You can't figure that 250 words will fit on a page because the client might want a three by five inch booklet. There will be photos and art work. You will have to calculate whether 100 words or less will go on each page. In this scenario, you can't submit a per-word rate. You need to ask for a flat fee.

If you are writing a booklet for a greeting card company, there might be 50 words on each page with plenty of art or advertising. Everything else will take up space, and the words will have to be few—perhaps 100, 50, or 25 words per page. This type of ghostwriting is similar to writing children's picture books where you write the story for the artist illustrating the book.

You're getting paid for your research. Therefore, it's necessary that you put as much information on paper as you'll need. Then organize it and pare down the words before you finish negotiations.

Where to Obtain a Degree

Contact University of the Sciences in Philadelphia • 600 South Forty-third Street • Philadelphia, PA 19104-44 for information on the following programs: Master of Science in Biomedical Writing, Regulatory Writing Certificate, Medical Marketing Writing Certificate or Professional development courses. USP offers Medical Writing programs leading to either a Master of Science in Biomedical Writing, or the various medical regulatory writing or medical marketing writing certificates.

The university's purpose in training medical writers is to, according to the department's Web site at: http://www.usip.edu/graduate/biomedwriting/ "to credential medical writers, to train medical writers to work ethically as professionals in private and public sectors of the healthcare industry, particularly the pharmaceutical industry to train pharmaceutical workers, life scientists and healthcare professionals to present ideas and data ethically and understandably.

The university's medical writing graduate degree and certificate programs are "are offered in blended online/onsite format with all instructors available by e-mail and telephone." The school makes all courses in medical writing available for remote students by offering onsite intensive courses during the summer semester.

Courses in the spring and fall semesters also have occasional onsite meetings on Saturday mornings and Monday through Thursday evenings. The department's students include those with graduate degrees in career transition, those who only want one or two courses. The Web site notes, "We occasionally accept exceptional recent graduates with twin interests in writing and life sciences."

According to the University of the Sciences, Philadelphia, PA, Biomedical Writing Curriculum Web site at: http://www.usip.edu/graduate/biomedwriting/curriculum.shtml, the core curriculum in biomedical writing for the MS degree in Biomedical Writing consists of the following courses:

Core Curriculum, Biomedical Writing

The curriculum for the Master of Science (MS) in Biomedical Writing consists of the following ten required courses (30 credits) plus six elective credits for a total of 36 credits:

BW701	Professional Writing in Science	3 credit hours
BW702	Stylistics and Editing	3 credit hours
BW703	Information Strategies for Biomedical Writers	3 credit hours
BW704	Regulatory Documentation Processes	3 credit hours
BW705	Biostatistics for Biomedical Writers	3 credit hours
BW706	Ethical and Legal Issues in Biomedical Communication	3 credit hours
BW860	Research in Biomedical Communication	3 credit hours
BW890	Graduate Research Project I	3 credit hours
BW891	Graduate Research Project II	3 credit hours

Students must take one of the following advanced regulatory writing courses:

BW707	Regulatory Writing: Medical Device Submissions	3 credit hours
BW708	Regulatory Writing: New Drug Applications	3 credit hours
Total Core Courses		30 credit hours
	Electives	6 credit hours
Total Curriculm Credits		36 credit hours

In addition, with the permission of the program director, students may enroll in complementary graduate courses at University of the Sciences in Philadelphia for credit in the biomedical writing program. Such courses are most likely to be offered by the university's graduate programs in Health Policy, Health Psychology, Pharmaceutical Business, or Pharmacy Administration. Students may also apply for transfer credits for graduate courses completed elsewhere.

Students with extensive experience in medical writing (5 or more years) may also seek the 'credit by examination' or 'life experience' option for required courses through formal application to the program director.

◆   ◆   ◆

What Ghostwriters-To-Be Need to Know

What you really need to know to become a medical ghostwriter is the basics of regulatory documentation, understanding statistics, and practice in writing a course for continuing medical education; a product monograph; a major research paper for publication; a website; and similar projects done daily at work as a medical ghostwriter or medical writer. You can learn the ropes and get the practice in several different ways.

The formal educational route is to take the graduate research projects courses and write the material learning hands-on as you go. Or you can take an internship with a company that lets you write or re-write and revise these documents for other writers.

For those who can't afford to take out loans to pay graduate school tuition, you can learn by reading books on these subjects, analyzing what you've read, and practicing writing the materials. Then put together a portfolio of samples that you've written. After all, students without graduate degrees in medical writing who have been medical writers for five or more years may take "credit by examination" or 'life experience' option for required courses. That means that there are employed medical writers and ghostwriters in the field who don't have a degree in medical writing and are still writing for pay. If this is your route, buy some books on biostatistics for biomedical writers and read them until you understand how to interpret data results.

Then buy some textbooks on regulatory documentation processes and writing and read those until you are able to begin practice writing the documents yourself. By joining professional associations for medical writers and biomedical editors, you can network, take seminars and continuing education courses given by the associations, attend meetings, work on newsletters, set up speakers panels at conventions, interview anyone who will talk to you at social gatherings (when they are not busy at work) and learn by practice, hands-on, through writing, revising, and re-writing until you have quality work to show in your portfolio.

Basically, what's required is good writing and knowledge of life sciences combined with regulatory processes and marketing documentation techniques. The cheapest way to prepare is by taking low-cost public community college courses divided half and half between journalism, English, marketing, public relations, advertising, and the biological sciences.

That's why community college graduates such as registered nurses who have had the courses in microbiology, anatomy, physiology, along with their nursing programs, pharmacy technicians, bioinformatics-genetics technology graduates, respiratory therapists, and other paraprofessional community college graduates can add a course in biostatistics.

Focus on seminars specifically for biomedical writers. Take some journalism courses such as advertising copywriting and science writing. Then transfer to a college for the last two years and finish a four-year degree in medical writing, life sciences, or journalism and communications with a science minor. With at least an undergraduate degree finished, you can get in the door of medical writing, and with some experience in a steady job, can finish your graduate degree in medical writing, sometimes at your employer's expense or on a part-time basis.

There are ways to save money and still be prepared. Medical writers are not licensed at the moment because the field is wide. Medical marketing writers focus on advertising and promotion in their writing. Regulatory medical writers are more science-focused on ghostwriting medical journal articles and regulatory reports. Both should have the same training, but the door into the field may have different experience requirements. Some medical writers enter the field from training in technical writing or science writing with a focus on a wide variety of sciences rather than emphasis on medicine. For example, schools offering master's degrees in science writing include, the University of Houston-Downtown. For their MS degree in Professional Writing & Technical Communication, see their Web site at: http://www.uhd.edu/academic/colleges/humanities/english/mspwtc.html.

What Do Regulatory Medical Writers Do?

Regulatory writers turn out what are referred to in the medical writing industry as GxP documents, which refers to "Good Laboratory, Clinical and Manufacturing Practices." A regulatory biomedical ghostwriter's job is about improving the quality and productivity of FDA-regulated activities. The writer clarifies language to explain standard operating procedures (called SOPs). Regulatory ghostwriters are supposed to help to improve compliance with Good Laboratory, Clinical and Manufacturing Practices (GxPs) by communicating complex scientific information in various GxP documents.

To prepare for a career in medical ghostwriting, you can either take a course in regulatory writing of GxP documentation or examine the process of writing GxP documents by analyzing those documents while you practice writing and editing those documents. The medical writing industry focuses on document writing of GLPs, which refers to Good Laboratory Practices, GCPs, which refers to Good Clinical Practices, and writing GMPs, which refers to Good Manufacturing Practices. When you lump GLPs, GCPs, and GMPs together, they are referred to in this industry as GxP documentation. Everything under this umbrella is referred to as regulatory writing.

Medical ghostwriters who do regulatory writing actually write regulatory documentation for biologic products of all types. To start to prepare on your own to be a medical ghostwriter, assuming you're choosing the autodidactic approach (teaching the trade to yourself instead of going to college for a graduate degree in biomedical writing), begin by examining the process of regulatory documentation. Some people like to learn independently.

They enjoy learning, but don't like school. Perhaps paying more than a thousand dollars per credit is not what you want to undertake at this time for a graduate degree in biomedical writing at some universities. You can do this on your own if you learn the same thing that the universities students are learning and create your own internships so you'll have hands-on practice.

Start first with learning about the FDA regulation of biological products. There are plenty of documents to read and research. You'll need to learn about the biological product development process by studying clinical documents. When you've re-read clinical documents and re-wrote them for practice, you'll start to practice communicating complex scientific information in a variety of documents.

Look at clinical studies. Analyze the ways the documents are edited, organized, and published. Proofread them. Look for issues unique to biological products. Talk to the vendors of the biological products and read their instructional literature. You'll find them at medical conferences, trade shows, events, expos, and conventions.

Tell them you're studying regulatory writing on your own to prepare for a career as a medical ghostwriter. Some of the more approachable regulatory writing available is about dietary supplements. Practice writing regulatory documentation for dietary supplements.

Read regulatory literature for dietary supplements. The FDA regulates dietary supplements. The FTC regulates dietary supplements. Read the documentation. Look at the FDA regulation of food additives. Read the complex scientific information. Look up the definitions and purchase a dictionary or glossary of scientific terms and a dictionary of medical terminology. Learn medical terminology. Focus in depth on issues unique to the type of regulatory documents you are studying.

How to Be a Ghostwriter in Continuing Medical Education

Continuing Medical Education (CME) is a growing area of specialization within biomedical writing. Ghostwriters develop CME courses by writing and designing effective CME programs in print and multimedia for all types of continuing medical education for consumers, nurses, therapists, technicians, physicians, pharmacists, dieticians, and any other occupation in the health care or medical industry. It's not only about writing the continuing education course material.

You have to understand how the approval process for running them is done. Contact publishers of continuing medical education programs and analyze how they are researched, put together, organized, written, edited, and published. Find out who buys the continuing medical education documentation and how they are used. You can set up your own entrepreneurial medical ghostwriting business with clients.

You can become a consultant. As an entrepreneur in medical ghostwriting, each time you'll approach a potential client, you'll need to write a mission statement, develop a business plan, and study legal, financial, and ethical issues of operating your own consultancy in biomedical communication. What you actually are is a biomedical communicator. You can enter this field as a journalist, medical sales representative in marketing, life science student or graduate, technical writer, or health care professional at any level from technician to physician, therapist to pharmacist. What you need is to get as much experience in medical writing as you can find.

◆   ◆   ◆

How to Be a Medical Marketing Writer

Promoting medical products also requires knowledge of FDA (Federal Drug Administration) regulations. Once you understand the FDA issues that affect medical marketing writers such as labeling documentation, you can move on to understanding the FTC (Federal Trade Commission) regulations covering promotion of biomedical products. Promotional writing techniques are similar to those in the copyrighting arena of advertising.

You have to communicate clearly complex scientific information in journal articles, CME (continuing medical education) posters, slide kits, and documents such as brochures, advertisements, and Web sites. Look at product labels and learn what FDA and FTC regulations are about concerning labeling of biomedical products, including food supplements.

Learn promotional writing techniques by looking pharmaceutical and medical product advertisements in direct-to-consumer publications. Compare the details in journal articles, magazines that are read mainly by physicians or other health care personnel to ads in medical newspapers.

Learning how to produce slide kits or brochures would be similar to what you learn in technical writing courses. You can look at how ads are put together to promote all types of technical information in various magazines. Read a book on promotional writing.

Document design is what you'll be doing most of the time to create text in a wide definition of words and illustrations. You don't need to spend thousands of dollars on a course to look at historical publications or attend lectures given by advertising and technical writing associations to listen to speakers discuss and demonstrate document design in print and digital media. But what you need to do is test your document to see whether it is effective and efficacious. What methods would you use for testing how effective your document is with your specific audience of scientists and physicians or pharmacists?

You'll have to ask those professionals whether your document is effective by showing them your promotional writing. Here's where an internship comes in handy where you can have contact, even in a professional association, with the medical professionals who read the publications where the promotional ads and illustrations, digital work, or photography appear.

Access and Balance Primary and Secondary Sources

The easiest way to become a medical ghostwriter is to read current health journal articles each week and write a report for practice. You need to increase your knowledge of disease, therapeutics, and medical products.

A course or good textbook in medical terminology helps. You can teach yourself medical terminology with a medical dictionary and a basic textbook if you do all the exercises in the book. You can find a used textbook on various used book sites online. An up-to-date book is what you want. Your goal is to gain facility in going to primary and secondary sources in equal numbers to find information about which to write. Look at writers' guidelines for medical journals and other medical publications.

Your purpose or goal is to understand how to write health care articles, reports, and promotional material such as advertising copy for the print media and digital markets. A wider scope is found with science writers, where the branch of science about which you'll write isn't restricted to medical products, continuing medical education, medical journal articles, regulatory reports, marketing materials, and pharmaceutical reports.

2. Where to Find Popular Clients or Publishers & Who Are Their Audiences?

Look for companies that produce reports, books, advertising copy, posters, learning materials, research, teaching, services, multimedia, or other materials in the fields of the following specializations, associations, nonprofits, publishing, or manufacturing industries:

Associations	Nephrology
Attention-Deficit/Hyperactivity Disorder	Nonprofits
Blood-Borne Illnesses	Neuro Medicine
Cardiology	Nutraceuticals
Consultants	Nutrition
Continuing Medical Education (CME)	Oncology
Dermatology	Ophthalmology
Drugs	Pain Management
Fundraisers	Pharmaceutical Manufacturers
Gastroesophageal Reflux Disease	Publishers
Genetics and Genetic Disorders	Radiology/Neuroradiology
Good Clinical Practices, GCPs	Regulatory Writing/Regulatory Agencies
Good Laboratory Practices, GLPs	Respiratory Diseases
Good Manufacturing Practices, GMPs	Rheumatology
Government	Sleep Disorders
GxP Documentation	Supplement Industry
Infectious Diseases	Therapists
Medical Devices	Think Tanks
Molecular Biology	Vaccines

◆   ◆   ◆

Look To Primary Sources Before You Look At Secondary Sources

Primary sources are better than secondary sources when you can find them. There's nothing like talking a little each day to a medical writing manager who has just retired and has time for informational interviews.

You can learn answers to the 100 questions following this segment through a variety of college or graduate level coursework or take seminars in any of these topics at most annual conferences of the American Medical Writers Association and/or similar organizations that offer continuing education in medical and/or science writing. Or you can research the answers on your own through reading documents and talking to experts and by asking for internships in documentation departments.

You don't need to have a science degree to belong to the American Medical Writers Association to break into medical writing, ghostwriting, or marketing journalism.

There are writers, editors, and indexers that are employed and/or that are members of national associations for medical writers that have degrees in a wide variety of subjects or no degree at all and are self-education.

These people do a wide variety of medical writing, editing, indexing, proof-reading, and other medical communication work. What they have in common is that they are biomedical communicators. Unlike nurses and physicians, medical writers do not need to be licensed or have to pass a national exam to find work in the documentation departments of corporations or nonprofits, regulatory document publishing, various agencies, or with publishers or marketing firms that produce medical devices, medicines, food supplements, or train professionals in continuing medical education.

Most corporations prefer someone with at least an undergraduate degree and writing experience. But once you work in medical writing, your experience is more important than your undergraduate degree major as long as you understand how to interpret biomedical information so that the people reading what you wrote approve.

Now that more universities are actually offering masters degrees in medical writing, it has become a respected career track standing by itself. No longer is medical writing a refuge for the bench scientist who wants to write or the technical writer who wants to do more than edit computer manuals or interview software engineers only to find the material is obsolete in three months.

Writing about clinical trails or medical journal articles offers adequate pay for the training spent. Biomedical ghostwriting gives you a purpose—making sure safety measures are in regulatory reports. You want to make sure that the negative effects as well as the positive ones are put into medical journal articles and reports on clinical trials sent to regulatory agencies. Medical ethics and conscience is at stake here for the ghostwriter.

You'll be researching, practicing, improving, and writing educational, scientific, or marketing material on the following medical communication themes: Here are 100 questions to ask experts in the field of medical ghostwriting so you'll know what you have to learn before you apply for a job as a medical ghostwriter.

Medical writers deal with macroediting and microediting issues and need to manage these issues. Microediting is selective editing. It is similar to your writing and editing being examined under a microscope to check for confusing sentences, weak points, flawed arguments, inconsistencies, and bad logic, errors in math, spacing, and correction of tables. In microediting, you need to validate and edit the item showing any changes from start to finish. You'd need to include historical information at micro-level. In order to find the historical information, for example, of a study from start to finish with applications and outcomes, you need to look at periodic surveys. For a great definition of microediting, macroediting, and copy editing, look at the American Medical Writers Association (AMWA) Journal, Volume 15, No. 4, page 19, Fall 2000. It's online at: http://www.amwa.org/default/publications/journal/v15.4/vol.15.no.4.p19.feature.pdf#search=%22macroediting%2C%20definition%22

Macroediting is editing the big picture. Most of what you'll do in medical ghostwriting is macroediting. You'd need to check for parallelism. You'd have to make sure various elements are parallel if they belong in the same series.

You'd make a list of graphs, figures, or tables. You'd check words for verb tense to make sure there were no inconsistencies or changes, and explain unfamiliar words. Copyediting of biomedical material consists of correcting language, format, and mechanical style to meet publication standards. You'd be required to do "substantive editing" and proofreading of your work at take charge of it by managing the editing process.

Biomedical ghostwriters use a particular style that makes the text unique to medical information, such as continuing education materials, advertising, or clinical trials and regulatory reports. You can teach yourself the stylistics of editing by reading the work of other medical writers who consistently produce good work.

There are principles of editing medial text and books on this subject to read. Start with the American Medical Association's *AMA Manual of Style*. Look for readability scales and grammar. Analyze medical text books and reports. You can form or join a medical writing critique group. If there's none nearby, create your own online. What you're looking for is to learn how to identify grammar and rhetoric while examining the trends in medical writing related to the *standards* of what is acceptable.

Medical writing has its own standards of what is correct. You need to understand what information you require and locate the sources. Then you should evaluate what information you find by searching medical, business, and government regulatory sources.

Learn how to use statistics for documentation.

When you are able to retrieve information as a freelance medical ghostwriter, not a university student, you'll have found the sources you need and obtained a freelance medical writer's permission documents or library card. Teach yourself to use biomedical information as a consultant or independent contractor and not as a student.

Focus on learning about regulatory documentation and the processes needed to write clinical and non-clinical design of research studies. What you're looking for specifically are regulatory reporting of a wide variety of biomedical products.

Biomedical research goes through specific procedures for which there are standardized formats for the various regulatory documents. You need to know the rules for submitting what you write such as the publication requirements, writers' guidelines, and other components necessary before you submit anything you write to any regulatory agency.

When you work as a medical ghostwriter, you'll be supervised by a medical writing manager. Find out what the manager has learned, perhaps by interviewing a recently retired medical writing department manager in the field of your choice—regulatory or marketing writing in the biomedical arena.

Convince your client or employer that microediting is what you are being paid to do even though much of your work would be macroediting or copyediting. You need to use exactly the right word without being too long-winded. Think of yourself as a "word plumber" administering "alternative editorial treatment" by looking at and comparing holistic and standard parts.

◆   ◆   ◆

101 Questions to Investigate about Medical or General Ghostwriting Techniques

1. What are good topics to write about concerning safety in workplaces or at home?

2. How do you write quality clinical summaries?

3. What's the best way to write or organize writing within very tight timelines?

4. What are the newest treatments for depression and suicidality?

5. How are macroediting and microediting handled?

6. How would a medical writer or editor handle critiques of biomedical research articles?

7. What is expected when analyzing and writing about sample size and Study Power? What are they about and how are they used in biomedical communications settings?

8. What types of outlining, punctuation, sentence structure, patterns, and proofreading techniques are used in medical ghostwriting to achieve maximum quality?

9. How is medical copyediting done? What emphasis or focus is expected when writing for an advertising or public relations agency with medical clients?

10. Where can grant proposal writing be learned and practiced in a short time?

11. What does medical journalism entail regarding choosing topics and polishing your writing?

12. How do you design and write patient education materials? (Excellent for those who have taught patients how to use equipment or medicine—such as registered nurses and various therapists—respiratory, physical, occupational, or dieticians, genetics counselors, psychologists, or other professional and/or

paraprofessional medical and health care personnel seeking a career switch into medical communications.)

13. What are the ethical standards used in medical communications?

14. How do you start freelancing?

15. How do you hire freelance medical ghostwriters through outsourcing to work for you in areas where they have the expertise but I don't have the training or experience my client wants?

16. What regulatory aspects of the drug develop process do I need to learn before I can ghostwrite clinical trials reports or medical journal articles?

17. What are the electronic regulatory submission rules I must learn?

18. Where can I learn to write clinical study reports so I can practice before I apply for a job?

19. What editorial processes do I need to learn before writing for medical journals?

20. What diseases should I write about that would attract the media's attention?

21. What is the best way to outline any type of medical writing?

22. How do I organize a biomedical paper? What are the rules?

23. How do I write abstracts, and what do I summarize as the big picture of a study?

24. Where can I review basic cell biology and microbiology for the nonscientist before applying for a job if I didn't have science courses in my journalism major?

25. How do I create attractive poster presentations that effectively hold the interest of physicians, scientists, and executives at medical conventions and conferences?

26. Where do I go to research drug interactions before I write any articles on clinical trials of drugs that will be sent to physicians and pharmacists?

27. What should I learn about writing electronic "common technical documents" and medical public relations materials?

28. Where can I learn about brain imaging? What are the best materials to read for the nonscientist writing for medical public relations firms?

29. What does it take to win government grants? What are they looking for in a document I will be asked to write?

30. What are employers looking for when they hire a freelance medical ghostwriter, and how much can I expect to earn? What must I learn or practice to earn maximum income? Do I need to have an advanced degree or be a physician or pharmacist, or can I climb the ladder as a freelance writer with a master's degree in medical writing?

31. What can be done to shorten the time it takes to outline, prepare, organize, and write excellent clinical study reports?

32. Is there money in freelancing on the topic of medical mysteries?

33. How do I attract and hold an audience with my writing style and substance? What does it take to be a catalyst?

34. What are the best strategies for improving the quality of the documents I write for the pharmaceutical industry?

35. What steps do I plan for in order to become a pharmaceutical communications manager?

36. How do I correct and revise flawed word usage (taxonomy) in medical writing?

37. How can learning basic medical terminology help me find a job as a medical ghostwriter?

38. What do I need to learn about statistics to become a medical writer?

39. How do I structure the patterns of my sentences in medical communications for clarity?

40. What are the best online databases I can search when practicing my medical writing?

41. What should I look for when proofreading?

42. What do I need to learn about epidemiology or basic anatomy to use in general medical communications?

43. How do I prepare CME materials?

44. What ethical issues must I learn before I can practice medical writing or ghostwriting?

45. What type of biomedical research design will I be working with as a medical writer?

46. What are the most important public relations techniques and materials I'll be using in medical marketing as a freelance writer?

47. How do I write an informed consent document?

48. How is the final report of a clinical trial written?

49. How do I push a document through a company's in-house reviewing process? What techniques will save time and yet focus on efficiency?

50. What words can I use to my advantage as a ghostwriter?

51. How do I best tailor my writing to my audience's needs?

52. How do I organize and write electronic regulatory submissions?

53. How do I edit grant proposals?

54. What is rhetorical grammar?

55. What size paragraphs are most effective in medical writing?

56. How do I launch a freelance medical ghostwriting career?

57. What's the editorial process like on medical and scientific journals?

58. What are the current trends in drug regulations?

59. How do I organize tables and graphs?

60. What are the latest updates on style manuals?

61. How can I design a newsletter that makes an impact?

62. What do I need to know about sample size?

63. What punctuation is required for the best clarity?

64. How do I deal with the big egos of scientists when I interview for primary sources? How can I tell when someone is approachable and respects medical writers?

65. What should I know about scientific integrity and honesty?

66. How do I deal with scientists whose corporations have a financial or conflict of interest in their trials?

67. How do I deal with regulators who have a financial interest or conflict of interest with the scientists' trials?

68. What kind of biomedical Web sites attract viewers?

69. How do I use Power Point and other methods for my slide kits and slide shows?

70. What's the best way to write great clinical summaries under pressure?

71. What's the best way to evaluate a medical writing contract?

72. What's direct-to-consumer advertising, and how does it change the way drugs are prescribed and public health?

73. What are the medical copyright do's and don'ts for a medical ghostwriter?

74. How are posters presented?

75. What should I know about medical discourse—entitlement and authority?

76. What are the most important pointers I should know as a medical marketing writer?

77. How do I know the difference between a high-quality clinical study and one that's not?

78. How do I get a job in health promotion?

79. What are the trends in disease prevention that a health promotion writer should know?

80. How can I best use my computer in medical literature searching?

81. How do I match syntax to rhetorical intent?

82. How do I report correlation and regression analyses if I've never had a course in statistics?

83. What sentence structure is best to use in medical ghostwriting?

84. What kind of journal submissions can I make other than research pieces?

85. What's the best way to turn research materials into articles?

86. How do I write popular articles on health or medicine for general consumer magazines?

87. What are the latest creative tips in pharmaceutical advertising copywriting?

88. How persuasively should I write?

89. How do I compose test questions that really are effective and efficacious?

90. Where do I find the medical information I need to write reports and articles?

91. How do I write a "final report" when I write a clinical trial report?

92. How do I write an investigator brochure?

93. If I'm asked to train or educate sales representatives, how do I customize my medical writing for sales people to understand and to make an impact?

94. How do I write indexes at the back of medical textbooks or continuing education books?

95. What types of issues will I be managing as a medical ghostwriter?

96. How do I write applications of investigational new drugs in a report?

97. How do I use creativity in biomedical writing?

98. When I transcribe a voice recording, how do I best edit the recording to get the most important facts? What should I leave in, and what should I cut?

99. How do I develop regulatory submissions when everyone I work with is working online from different cities?

100. What's the best way to develop a manuscript from start to submission?

101. How do I prepare clinical study protocols for peer review when I'm under tight time constraints? What electronic methods for confirming documentation can I use to cut wasted time?

◆   ◆   ◆

3. How to Get an Assignment

Check out the employment needs of the larger pharmaceutical firms and medical publications. As daily newspapers and general consumer magazines merge or downsize, specialty publications increase in diversity of topics to meet readers' needs. Look at the latest job openings list at the Web site of the American Medical Writers Association. You need to be a member.

Also join or attend meetings of a variety of science writers and biomedical editors' associations. There's a list of associations at the back of this book in the appendix.

Before you join an association, attend a meeting and network with the people to find out whether this is the career you want to pursue. Also contact the editorial departments of medical publications such as newspapers, newsletters, and magazines to find out submission guidelines. Learn the difference between a medical journal and a general consumer magazine that prints feature articles on medical topics, healthcare, or medical economics. You might also join the Association of Healthcare Journalists. The association's Web site is at: http:// www.ahcj.umn.edu/. The difference between a medical ghostwriter or medical writer and a healthcare journalist is that the healthcare journalist may not necessarily have had any formal training in medical writing or in healthcare and may be a general assignment reporter on a newspaper or magazine who writes health care-related features, fillers, and articles for general consumer publications such as daily newspapers or more generalized magazines read by the public.

Medical writers may write for regulatory agencies and physicians. But medical writers may also write for general magazines. Generally, a healthcare journalist does not write heavily technical material, but gears the journalism to the general public. See the O'Sullivan's Writing Classes Medical Writing Resources List on the Web at: http://www.maryfo.com/mfo/general_resources/technical/medical.htm. Also online, see the Health Sciences Journals resource list at the University of Washington at: http://depts.washington.edu/hsic/journals/. Search the Librarians' Index to the Internet for Health and Medicine for more resources at: http://lii.org/search/file/health.

Of course, medical writers and health care journalists may write for one another's publications at different times, and either may write medical marketing articles. But medical writers are more likely to write clinical trials reports and regulatory materials or medical journal articles, usually ghostwritten. Healthcare journalists usually write for the general public under their own bylines.

4. How to Hone Training and Specialize

You can specialize in general ghostwriting for public relations and corporate environments or in an area of specialty such as medical regulatory or marketing, or any other subject—legal for instance if you have a legal or paralegal background. Other areas could be finance, current affairs, women's issues, psychology, art, music, or any other specialization.

Ghostwriters are frequently hired in the medical, pharmaceutical, and health care fields because of the wide need for patient and medical continuing education materials in text and digital formats. There's also a need for writing clinical trials reports, regulatory information, and advertising for medical, scientific, and technical products.

Specialize and hone your training in one area where there is an increasing demand for ghostwriting. Right now that field is medicine and pharmaceutical products. Ten years ago the 'in' field was high technology—software manuals and instructional technical writing. There also is opportunity in educational writing. If you teach a specialty subject, focus on your area of training. If that area is not in demand for ghostwriters, find an allied field that you can transfer your skills to and add more education or training so you have expertise in writing about a field that is in high demand, such as marketing and promoting of specific products through copywriting.

5. Ghostwriting Books, Proposals, and Query Letters

Prepare your portfolio by developing sample book proposals and query letters. Write three chapters of a book manuscript that you'll use as a sample. Query literary agents and publishers of specialty books as well as managers or agents of celebrities. If you want to be a ghostwriter, select a niche in the area of your expertise. If you're a generalist, then approach publishers and literary agents as well as the marketing communications departments of larger corporations. Generalist ghostwriters get their start by editing manuscripts or by writing articles for busy professionals in the corporate world. You could specialize in speechwriting or writing regulatory reports in fields outside of medicine.

You could write instructional manuals and focus on technical writing or approach the managers and agents of celebrities and their public relations agents with your brochure on ghostwriting life stories or material on special topics. Create your own niche.

You could open a ghostwriting business where you fish out assignments to other ghostwriters in the medical or legal field while you specialize in your own niche or remain a generalist. Another area of focus is ghostwriting memoirs. But it is more difficult to maintain stead work by writing memoirs of people willing to pay. It's easier to ghostwrite medical articles or regulatory reports and advertising copy for the larger pharmaceutical firms.

6. Ghostwriting Speeches

Let your local chamber of commerce and convention bureau know you ghostwrite speeches. Inform professional associations and employee newsletters, large corporations—marketing communications departments, political parties and candidates, professionals such as physicians and attorneys, teachers, executives, and public relations agencies, publishers, authors, and government that you ghostwrite speeches.

Talk to medical firms, the media, PTA, school boards, universities, librarians, events planners, speakers' bureaus, party planners, and various houses of worship. Speeches are given not only by members of speakers' associations and speakers' bureaus, but by those who set up speakers' panels for conferences. Contact groups, clubs, and organizations, including the nonprofits and the fundraisers.

7. Ghostwriting Booklets or Brochures

In general ghostwriting, booklet writing usually comes out of corporations' marketing communications and public relations departments. With medical writing, continuing medical education and patient education may be put into booklets, digital instruction, or brochures.

Most public relations and advertising firms associated with the larger pharmaceutical firms use medical marketing writers. Outside of medical ghostwriting, booklets or brochures are used by vendors and publishers, for training, and with instructions included with product packaging. Societies for technical writers, trainers, and teachers also are helpful if you write instructional materials.

8. Copywriting is Ghostwriting

Most advertising copywriting is ghostwriting. No one puts a byline on an advertisement, unless it's the illustrator's signature. The marketing department of a large pharmaceutical firm is the place to show your medical marketing copywriting skills. Create a portfolio of advertisement copy to show as a sample.

Also try the marketing communications departments, advertising agencies, and associations for copywriters and editors. You can also join biomedical editors associations or marketing associations at the national level and work on the job leads for your local chapter.

9. Ghostwriting Newsletters

Design your own sample newsletters with software templates. Put your samples on the Web to show and on a CD or DVD disc. Most firms have employee newsletters. Talk to the public relations, publications, and marketing communications departments of almost any large corporation.

For medical ghostwriting of newsletters, focus on the medical and consumer publishers and the medical economics publications. Research databases of what firms have their own employee newsletters that use outsourced help or have openings for communications managers or staff and freelance writers, editors, or proofreaders. Also talk with printers whose clients may be hiring people to write newsletter material or design templates for digital content.

10. Coaching For Key Topics

Ghostwriters can use coaching from people who work in the type of industries that frequently hire medical ghostwriters—which is the pharmaceutical industry and manufacturers of medical products from gadgets surgically implanted to food supplements. The best way to get coaching is to take a seminar given by a professional association or university or attend conventions and conferences. Or you can volunteer to work on the newsletter of a professional association. The next best way to get coaching is to ask for an internship with a large pharmaceutical firm in their publications or communications department.

If you want to be a coach, print up your brochures, booklets, and business cards, and start a group or a class in teaching others how to be ghostwriters by calling experts to speak on a panel or at a monthly meeting of your group. Another way is to write for publications in the field you want to enter or volunteer to set up speakers' panels at conventions and conferences. Work closely with publicists, marketing communications managers, and events planners whether you want to coach or be coached in ghostwriting marketing. Another niche is writing success stories and case histories or life stories of people in the public arena. There are government jobs open from time to time in the regulatory divisions. Keep applying and preparing for these types of jobs. In the meantime, work as an independent contractor and freelance your ghostwriting skills to publishers and literary agents, physicians' or attorneys' groups, and corporate communications marketing departments.

11. Working with Publicists and Public Relations Directors

Join various local chapters of national public relations societies and network with people in public relations. Write for public speakers or speak yourself to let others know that you ghostwrite for their clients.

Show your portfolio of samples to marketing communications managers of corporations, hospitals, pharmaceutical firms, and publishers. Join technical writing societies and look at their job leads. To ghostwrite life stories for celebrities, contact their managers, agents, or publicists. Ask the owners of public relations agencies that represent celebrities or publish books about them to assign you a book to ghostwrite for the agency or for one of the celebrities.

12. How Long Does it Take to Ghostwrite a Book?

A non-fiction ghostwritten book of 70,000 words generally takes six months to write. You can specialize in how-to books, current issues, medical, scientific, or technical material, instructional, or fiction. A romance novel of 24 chapters can take anywhere from six months to a year to research and write. A non-fiction book usually takes less time to write than fiction, depending up the type of research.

Career development books usually take three to six months. You can write a book on home repair, for example, in six months to a year. Or you can spend a year ghostwriting a memoir or life story of a celebrity or executive because the information would have to be approved and revised several times. Medical books have to be microedited to make sure there are no inconsistencies or inaccurate information and that the research is current.

13. Working on a Per-Word Rate

If there are a few words to write, such as 50 words on a greeting card or 100 words on a brochure, charge three dollars per word. If there are many words, charge a flat fee, since you won't get any royalties, the person whose name is on the book as the author will get the royalties. Work out with your agent or publisher what the flat fee will be.

Put it in writing in your contract along with the due date. Have a literary properties attorney look at your contract to make sure you don't have to pay your agent expenses for things such as foreign rights, phone bills, copying costs, and postage. For magazine articles, you may get more like one or two dollars per word, depending upon the magazines, but for greeting cards, three dollars per word for 50 words is acceptable. Ask other ghostwriters what they are getting and average it out for your neck of the woods.

Anytime you're writing a booklet or book where there are many words, charge a flat fee, say $10,000 or $100,000, depending upon what you are being paid to write and research. Is a think tank's research and surveys behind your own research? If the author assigned to write an article is being paid $1 a word and hires you to ghostwrite a magazine article, you'll probably get more like 50 cents a word.

You can also charge a per-word rate to ghostwrite academic papers, but it isn't ethical to write someone else's thesis and will eventually be found out. Most legitimate ghostwriting is done by medical and pharmaceutical firms hiring knowledgeable, experienced ghostwriters to write articles for medical journals or regulatory commissions

Writing, macroediting, and microediting are based on careful research from clinical trials. Of course, there are numerous articles online where the ghostwriters don't have medical doctor (MD) degrees.

Some medical journal articles have been criticized in the media for having emphasized the positive results and having not included any negative results, but before you accept *opinion* from various media articles online, check out and investigate the facts behind the opinions. Do the facts speak volumes? Investigate for yourself before you begin a career as a medical or any other type of ghostwriter or editor.

Think for yourself. Investigative reporting is needed in the medical field. What studies are flawed? What's the credibility of those who point out flaws? Talk to ghostwriters and see whether or not they are qualified to write those types of articles. Who watches the watchers? Then decide for yourself. Learn the difference between opinion and fact and check facts carefully. Your knowledge is based on your own microediting.

14. Designing a Budget Template

If you want to open your own ghostwriting business, design a template for your budgets. Before you are hired by a client, you'll need templates of sample budgets to show how much you'll need for each step of the ghostwriting process.

Keep a laminated page in your portfolio or loose leaf binder with a separate template for each type of budget you'll need to make for sample companies. The mock-up you'll make will be to show clients how you will spend the money you're given to ghostwrite a particular project such as a report, article, booklet, brochure, instructional script, or book.

15. Ghostwriting for Entertainment Celebrities

It pays in contacts to attend conferences where the owners of public relations and advertising agencies attend, such as the various small press publishers associations. Talk to the managers and agents of celebrities in the entertainment, music, or political professions about your ghostwriting work. Show samples.

Put your work on CDs or DVDs and other digital forms as well as print formats. Write to the agents of celebrities and to the celebrities with your brochure and business card. Send one great sample of your work. Offer to write biographies of your favorite celebrities and send your query letters to publishers of books and booklets on the life stories of your favorite celebrities. Do the same for celebrities who straddle entertainment, politics, music, or corporate environments in the field of your choice, such as business or health.

16. Ghostwriting for Professionals: Medical, Legal, Scientific, Political, Academic, Literary Authors, and Others.

The quickest way to let specialists know that you ghostwrite books about them or their subject of expertise is to write them and their agents, publishers, or managers. Anyone can write an unauthorized biography and contend with the fuss when and if the book is published.

To write an approved, ghostwritten book you need to go through the protocols of their employers, agents, managers, or public relations representatives. Often, you start with the marketing communications department of their corporations. Not all ghostwritten books are life stories of the rich and famous. Some ghostwritten books are academic or textbooks meant for university instruction. Some ghostwritten books bear the names of professors or students, and some the names of medical celebrities.

You can start collecting names from speakers' bureaus to see whether any of the professional public speakers want books or booklets or even articles ghost-written about their work. Sometimes public speakers prefer to speak rather than to write. You may end up transcribing their recorded voices or taking oral history and transcribe it into text to be archived in oral history libraries.

17. Ghostwriting and Simplifying Different Types of Speeches

Ask speakers' bureau representatives and members whether they would like to have you ghostwrite speeches. Also contact political parties' headquarters, candidates, corporate executives, vendors at conventions, and publishers. Find out who gives lots of speeches and whether you can write the speeches. Various comprehensive health planning agencies and nonprofit agencies, fundraisers, and event planners can use someone to write speeches that someone else will give.

You don't have to be a public speaker yourself to write speeches that another person will deliver to the public. You need to be a writer of vivid words. Play back everything you write and record digitally. You need to know how your writing sounds to the ear to get the timing and rhythm of the speech right. Ask others to listen to any recordings of speeches you write and get feedback on what kind of impact the words make. Are your words memorable? Why?

18. Researching Speeches & Speakers' Bureaus: International & National

Write to speakers' bureaus around the world focusing on those whose members and executives speak any language you know well. Attend seminars, conventions, and conferences as well as teleconferences. Find out who is presenting or shows up on a panel. Ask whether that person's corporation hires speech writers.

Speakers' bureaus may have a requirement that each speaker make a minimum amount per year from speaking, such as $2,000 or more in pay for each speaking engagement. The speakers' bureau requirements differ. Contact professional associations that have speakers' bureaus.

19. Audio-Visual & Multimedia Speechwriting & Ghostwriting Techniques

Familiarize yourself with how to put your ghostwriting samples in multimedia format, such as on DVDs, CDs, or Web sites. If you ghostwrite continuing medical education materials or any type of how-to or instructional material for trainers or students, you'll need to make the material interactive to some degree.

Obtain the software you need to transfer your writing to digital format and present your brochures, booklets, book chapter samples or articles in print and electronic format. One creative idea is to make your brochure round or oval in shape so that a pocket for a CD or DVD at the back carries what is in print also in digital form with video clips or illustrations and photos.

20. Ghostwriting Memoirs & Autobiographies

If you only want to ghostwrite memoirs, research people who have enough money to pay you a flat fee to write their life stories or experiences. If the person is a celebrity, work through the literary agent, book publicist, publisher, or public relations and marketing communications departments of their employer.

If the person is not a celebrity, find out who represents them to the media. Have the agent, entertainment or literary rights attorney draw up a contract whereby you will be paid a flat fee in thirds—one third upon signing, one third when half way through, and the final third when the manuscript is done and in the hands of the publisher.

Usually the publisher or literary agent or a literary/entertainment attorney draws up the contract. If you want to have the book auctioned to the highest bidder—usually a publisher or sometimes an agent, contact an entertainment or literary rights attorney that usually represents authors and publishers.

The best way to find celebrities is through their agents, managers, employers, or publishers. But you can still write to them at their business address and send a query letter with your business card and brochure of your work as a ghostwriter.

21. Using Humor in Ghostwriting

Well-written humor makes an impact. Use it where it works best.

Ask your client where it is appropriate to use humor in a ghostwritten article, book or booklet. It's not appropriate in a medical report, but in a general magazine, humor works to introduce a topic if it has the element of surprise. Ask other ghostwriters to send you their most humorous experiences as ghostwriters. Then ask ghostwriters what was the most important lesson they learned from life as a ghostwriter. Making full use of what you have is a frequently quoted answer in the media—reaching your potential.

22. Ghostwriting Scripts, Skits, Plays and Monologues from Current Issues

Most ghostwriting is in book format. Some ghostwriting of scripts is done by experienced or retired scriptwriters known to the industry where they worked previously. Educational and industrial scripts often are ghostwritten. Contact the media department of a corporation with your samples of training or industrial scripts you want to ghostwrite for the corporation's marketing communications, training, or public relations departments.

You may want to ghostwrite training scripts in continuing medical education or any other type of on-the-job training or how-to instruction. Making documentaries on your own helps you to get the experience you'll need in writing non-fiction scripts for corporations. The sure way in is to ask for an internship in the audio-visual media department of a corporation where the training and product demonstration videos are made.

If you're more interested in writing life stories in play or script format, contact the agents and managers or publishers of the people you want to portray in script form. If the celebrity or scholar is long gone, the publisher of the individual's works is the department to contact—the permissions department of a publisher. To learn how to write the scripts, check out the book titled, *How to Write Plays, Monologues, or Skits from Life Stories, Social Issues, or Current Events: For All Ages* by Anne Hart Pages: 238, ISBN: 0-595-31866-5, Published: May-2004.

23. Media Connections

Launch news releases of about one page in length or brief filler articles about yourself as a ghostwriter in the media if you want others to know you do ghostwriting for a flat fee or on a per-word basis. Send these brief pieces to magazines and daily newspapers as well as niche newspapers such as ethnic publications, industrial trade journals and industrial newsletters.

Join press clubs and let reporters know you do ghostwriting for clients, either on your own as an independent contractor or on the staff of a corporation. The companies that use long-term, steadily employed ghostwriters are mostly the larger pharamaceutical firms, the giants, and similar types of medical corporations.

The easiest way to reach these firms is by looking them up in library corporate databases to get names and addresses or joining a medical writer's organization and looking at the job referrals online or in the newsletters mailed to members.

If you don't want to spend money yet to join a professional association, most university libraries have a business division where you can look up names and addresses of the various corporations and send your query letters to their publications departments. Instead of wasting time asking for informational interviews that busy executives under time pressure won't give unless they know you, send a brochure with a sample report or article, brochure or booklet either in print and/or digitally on disc so they know that your writing is what they need at the moment. Some ghostwriters also do job coaching or public speaking.

It's better to specialize and emphasize one area of expertise you want to ghostwrite in, such as medial marketing or regulatory ghostwriting. If you don't want to ghostwrite for the medical markets, then choose an area in which you have expertise and in which there is a need for ghostwriting on a steady basis.

If you rely on making money by writing the life stories of the rich and famous, you're in for competition from the publicists who manage those celebrities and the employees or outsourced talent of those publicists. If you work with the marketing communications department of a corporation or its advertising agency, you'll need a portfolio of all the types of ghostwriting you do expertly. See the article by D. Zuckerman titled, *Hype in health reporting: "checkbook science" buys distortion of medical news. International Journal of Health Services.* 2003;33(2).

24. Ghostwriting Styles

Your style depends upon the type of ghostwriting you do. Medical ghostwriting uses styles different from general ghostwriting of non-technical, non-scientific materials. You can buy a book on writing styles such as *The Elements of Style* by William Strunk, Jr. Or read the book online at Bartleby.com Great Books Online at: http://www.bartleby.com/141/.

Your publisher will tell you what style to follow and usually will recommend a book that tells you how to use a particular style of writing for a particular type of publication. Buy a classic reference book that's related to the type of ghostwriting you select.

For medical ghostwriting, try the *American Medical Association Manual of Style*, 9th edition. Baltimore, MD et al.: Williams & Wilkins, 1998. Contact information: www.wwilkins.com, 800-638-0672. Also read *Medical English Usage and Abusage*. Edith Schwager (AMWA member), Phoenix, AZ, Oryx Press, 1991. Contact information: www.greenwood.com, 800-225-5800. See Appendix

C for a list of books that help your writing styles if you choose medical writing. For general ghostwriting, choose a book on language usage, editing, and writing styles closest to the area of your expertise.

1

Popular Health & Medical Writing for Magazines

How to Turn Current Research & Trends into Salable Ghostwriting or Feature Articles

Making Medical Language Specialists
Turning Medical Transcribers into Medical Writers & Editors

Consumer health, medical, and pet magazine editors are more interested in new trends rather than broad-based stories. Technical and medical writing skills can move a medical transcriber to an editor's or reporter's job with a publisher of medical or medical economics publications or with a public relations agency. You won't be able to get a job writing medical reports or journal articles if you are a medical transcriber with a basic high-school education, but with course work in medical writing, doors begin to open.

With an undergraduate degree in medical writing and editing, you can make it to the public relations department, a medical news publication, or editing, indexing, and proofreading medically-oriented books. Or you could continue your education to become a medical librarian or medical language teacher or trade journal reporter or editor.

If you earn a masters' degree in biomedical writing and editing or medical marketing writing, you can apply for jobs in the documentation division of large pharmaceutical firms, with government agencies, and with nonprofits or open your own medical ghostwriting service and outsource other medical writers with different types of degrees and specializations. It's one way to have your own business. Another direction would be to ask for an internship in medical writing or ghostwriting with a pharmaceutical or medical products corporation.

A different writing or editing career possibility is to become a technical writer/editor/indexer/proofreader and specialize in one area of technical writing such as indexing medical textbooks. Community colleges offer degrees in technical communications. Another field is traveling to conventions and conferences to design and create medical newsletters or summarize what was presented at the conferences for a newsletter or medical newspaper. Medical economics publications also use writers with good verbal skills to report on the business end of a medical, pharmaceutical, or dental practice. You could also work on continuing medical education course materials and make use of your knowledge of medical terminology and correct grammar.

Medical transcribers, medical record administrators, and medical case history writers, librarians, indexers, editors, interpreters, and proofreaders are medical language specialists. Language specialists can become writers, editors, or indexers. They can become book packagers and information brokers. What it takes is learning the ability to turn technical and scientific terms into plain language for a general consumer and audience. Write for general magazines and trade journals. Focus on trends or magazine journalism.

Learn to research articles and interview experts. Here's how to transform your medical terminology knowledge, listening ability, and keyboarding skills into interviewing, researching, and explaining clearly for people with non-technical backgrounds what new findings are out there that concern the reader's well-being.

If in the future, medical transcribers will be replaced by computers that take technical dictation and transcribe correctly all accents, your highly developed listening and medical language specialist skills could be transformed into administrative or editorial record maintenance work. You could go in several directions: medical record administration and coding, research, editing, sales of transcribing software and equipment, or medical journalism.

For those who always wanted to write or edit medical publications, scripts, medical record histories, case histories, or books, here's a guide to becoming a medical writer or editor. For those interested in video, you could write and produce medical videos by interviewing experts on camera or by working behind the scenes to produce medical or self-help videos (on DVDs).

Medical, healthcare, and science or technical writers and editors (who have some skills similar to transcribers) earned a median annual salary of $37,400, had a 23 percent (long term—11-year) job growth rate, an excellent short-term outlook, excellent job security rating, an average prestige rating, and a low-stress and strain rating, according to <u>Money</u> magazine's March 1994 job rankings article.

Currently, the growth rate is still in effect. Technical writers ranked number 18 out of 100 occupations ranked as "The Best Jobs in America." (Their sources included the Bureau of Labor Statistics.) <u>Money</u> also stated that the best places to work in this kind of job are Silicon Valley, Boston, or Washington, DC.

How giant a leap is it for a medical transcriber (earning an average of $15,000 to $30,000 after ten to twenty years on the job) to transfer good language skills and advance to a career in biomedical communications—to any one of the following medical publications professional job titles where salaries of more than $30,000 can be reached without having to be on the same job for decades?

Jobs in medical journalism include researching trends, medical marketing, videography, and the following print or electronic editorial positions:

Medical journalist, science writer, medical copyeditor, technical writer/editor, publications proofreader, scientific publication coordinator, pharmaceutical copywriter, documentation analyst, hospital grant proposal writer and fundraising publicist/press release writer, trade journal reporter/stringer, health communications publicist, medical desktop publisher, desktop video producer, vocational teacher, corporate trainer, medical communications public speaker, newsletter and publications designer, medical sales direct mail marketing writer, medical textbook editor, back-of-book and periodical indexer, medical journal article abstractor, member of the medical, computer, or scientific press, on-line (computerized) medical editing service entrepreneur, medical radio scriptwriter, health video training scriptwriter, infomercial writer/producer, niche publisher, abstractor, or freelance medical communications coordinator/writer/editor combination.

Any one of these professional jobs requires the same language skills every medical transcriber has, plus a flair for creative expression in print or electronic media. Therefore, if you are tired of typing all day, tired of having your keystrokes and bathroom breaks electronically monitored, and tired of carpal tunnel syndrome surgery, or if you are far enough over fifty to place less emphasis on high speed typing and more on creativity and intuition enhancement—perhaps you'd like to become a medical writer, editor, or publications coordinator.

Some medical transcribers have liberal arts degrees or college coursework in English, communications, journalism, or professional writing and editing or education. Others have two-year community college degrees in health information technology management or in medical transcription.

Numerous medical transcribers have language or English teaching credentials and are re-entering the workforce after taking time out to raise a family. Others are laid-off workers from other fields, including newspaper reporting.

In this semester's beginning medical transcription class at Grossmont College in El Cajon, CA, at least one student had a master's degree in a foreign language and another had a master's degree in English and was a fulltime freelance writer. At Mesa College's medical terminology class, this semester, more male students were beginning a course of study in preparation for careers as medical transcribers.

One male student with a college degree in architectural drafting who was changing careers to medical transcription said he enrolled because he has a wife and children to support and thought that medical transcription would provide a better chance of finding employment and job security. More males are coming into the field this year, at least in San Diego.

At the same time, a lot of more mature women seeking more of a career in less of a job market are taking courses in medical terminology and transcription. Some are coming from the ranks of college graduates with degrees in English and professional writing.

Those with these degrees are seeking road paths to advancement using their medical terminology skills. After taking courses in terminology, anatomy and physiology, pathophysiology, and advanced medical transcription, these students with degrees in humanities are using the training to seek jobs in medical writing and editing.

They're finding jobs by joining professional and trade associations and advertising in the trade journals or answering the ads in the job "hot sheets." The organizations they're joining include The American Medical Writers Association, The National Association of Science Writers, The Council of Biology Editors, Freelance Editorial Association, National Association of Writing Consultants, American Association of Journalists and Authors, and other organizations (addresses appear at end of this article).

Being a medical language specialist means having the option to advance when you want to from transcriber to editor or writer. With the advent of voice recognition computers, more medical transcription work will be directed to editing and proofreading—such as using the American College of Physicians and Surgeons guidelines to prepare the articles of scientists and physicians to meet the editorial requirements and standards of the majority of medical and scientific journals.

What Does A Medical Writer Do?

A variety of jobs exist for medical writers depending upon whether you work for a biotechnical industry company doing molecular genetics research or gene-splicing and DNA experiments, or whether you work for a biomedical firm which manufactures and sells medical instruments and equipment, software, or medical and hospital supplies.

In a pharmaceutical manufacturing firm, an ad copywriter works in-house in the advertising, public relations, or marketing communications department writing drug advertisements for brochures on the newest drugs sent or directed to physicians and medical journal advertisements. The copywriters also work closely with the art department to design brochures and the material that accompanies prescription drugs, the writing on the packaging, and direct mail marketing literature going to physicians and hospitals.

In a hospital, the medical writer may write grant proposals for a new building, new MRI imaging system, or other needs as well as proofread literature published by the hospital for the doctors or for patient education pamphlets and other literature.

Some medical communicators are hired to be "go-getters" in order to make calls, do fundraising (find money), and write other material accompanying grant proposals for further funding of new or existing projects of a medical or community nature.

Where Jobs Are

Jobs for medical writers and editors exist in medical publishing with book publishing houses or with the medical newspaper and trade journal press going to physicians or allied healthcare personnel. Freelance medical writers for trade journals telephone professionals such as respiratory therapists, nurses, physicians, and physical therapists, ask much focused questions (such as all the steps the therapist uses to teach patients how to use and clean respiratory therapy equipment).

After interviewing a variety of professionals by phone, the interview is taped through a telephone recording device. The medical writer transcribes the article, editing out wordiness and redundancy. The article is finally whittled down to the 2,000 or 3,000 words the publisher usually requires.

In an oral interview, there is a lot of skipping around, so the article must be organized. Each subject is cut and pasted by computer in categories. Like subjects are grouped together. Finally, the article is polished, proofread, edited, and checked for organization and active verbs. Sentences are shortened to about 10 to 15 words each, and a hook lead is put at the beginning to attract and keep the attention of the reader.

A medical article directed to physicians may go through several iterations, revisions and copyediting, then checked once more with the experts for accuracy.

Unlike a home based transcriber left alone with a tape, the home based freelance writer, editor, or staff reporter can always pick up the phone and ask the doctor to clarify facts or explain technical material for an audience of general readers or allied health workers from other fields, including nursing and technology.

The article is finally checked for its ability to stick to the subject and provide information for the reader to use to make professional decisions. Most medical articles are written for other medical professionals or technicians as readers. The freelance writer for healthcare publications read by the public is written in a clear-to-understand news style like a popular magazine or newspaper article, following the publisher's guidelines.

Medical textbook editors are hired for their ability to copyedit manuscripts written by professionals. The grammar and spelling are clarified, according to the publisher's style. Medical book indexers create indexes at the back of medical books, periodical indexers index medical journal, magazine, and newsletter publications, and journal abstractors summarize in 200 words or less, the important information extracted from medical journal articles for library directories, reference books, and research periodicals.

Jobs for communicators, editors, and writers—with knowledge of medical terminology—are available in medical school libraries and public affairs offices. You're not limited to being a transcriber, coder/indexer, tumor registrar, or a records administrator/technician, particularly if you have an artistic or creative flair with medical language and a need to express yourself in print or electronic media.

The Job of the Biomedical Publications Coordinator

The hospital publications coordinator edits and coordinates the production of a variety of publications from concept through design, pre-press, printing, and distribution. A publications coordinator working in a hospital or medical school teaching facility earns an average of $2,300 to $2,700 monthly.

You don't need a four-year degree to coordinate publications. A two-year degree in technical writing, journalism, English, health information management technology, or transcription plus a few short journalism, writing, proofreading and editing courses taken at your local university's extended studies department is helpful, but not required.

The best experience is on-the-job or through volunteer work at medical meetings open to journalists. Volunteer on the publications of professional associations, hospitals, research institutes, and medical schools. Ask what you can do for your medical trade journals, volunteer at conferences in the press room or on the public relations team of the organization putting on the conference or medical convention.

Skills required include the ability to proofread, copyedit, and correct text for accuracy, clarity, punctuation, grammatical and syntactical correctness and continuity. The publications coordinator is responsible for written articles, coordinating the receipt of articles by other authors, and working with graphic artists to develop design and layout.

The publications coordinator works independently, copyediting and proofreading all publications that come out of the institution. Editing and writing is done on brochures, newsletters, policy papers, and conference volumes.

Skills needed are the same as for a transcriber, minus the constant high-speed keyboarding. The work is more varied and a lot more creative.

Medical writing is both an intellectual and creative outlet if you're the artistic or literary type of person with a focus on medical communications, mental health information dissemination, or observing and reporting the news on new advances in molecular genetics, epidemiology, biology, medical software, medical economics, advertising and publicity, or pharmacy and the consumer.

It's for the investigative type person also, interested in working in health promotion communications, pathology, radiology, or medical training communications and multimedia instructional design for training healthcare personnel. Or perhaps you'd like to write about the home health care industry and broadcast or share the news.

You'll do a lot of proofreading, copyediting, and correcting text for accuracy. You'll need excellent narrative skills for writing press releases to announce new products. In a hospital setting or in a research institute, writing may be done for the publicity department or for the manager of internal communications.

The Work of the Publications Coordinator Offers Variety

The publications coordinator writes speeches that physicians give at conferences. You'll need creative skills in planning the layout of various materials such as flyers, newsletters, book covers (book jackets).

You may even help plan for events, medical trade shows, conferences, press and scientific meetings, seminars, and conventions or work in public relations. Or you may be assigned to be a documentation analyst, production editor, or liaison between the graphic design, courseware design, and editorial departments.

If you can conceptualize production schedules for publications from start to finish and coordinate all steps involved, you have the qualifications to become a publications coordinator. You'll need strong computer word-processing skills, desktop publishing skills, a knowledge of how graphic arts work together with text, a knowledge of how databases work (for retrieval using databases), and word-processing applications. You'll need familiarity with concepts and medical or scientific terminology in your field of choice.

Education or Training for Writing Careers?

The kind of education you'll need for this generalist type of job is the equivalent of advanced education in English, Journalism, communications, or public relations/advertising copywriting, or a combination of education and experience or self-learning in an editorial function and medical terminology.

You can get this type of training by taking an adult school or community college journalism course, by reading yourself, taking a correspondence course in journalism or copyediting, or asking a journalism professor to give you a reading list in how to copyedit or report medical news. Try volunteering in the information or public relations department or work on the newsletter of your local medical school, teaching or county hospital, pharmaceutical manufacturing company, or biomedical research institute.

Learning On the Job, Through Internships, Or By Volunteering

If you join the American Medical Writers Association, core courses are given at conventions that will help you make the transition from transcriber to medical writer/editor. It's not an absolute necessity to pursue a four-year degree in the humanities.

It's better to get experience as a freelance writer or editor on publications where you can volunteer your time or serve an internship. Ask your local professional organization if you can volunteer to work on a newsletter, trade association journal, or magazine doing editing and writing.

It's still possible to be an autodidact. Teach yourself medical writing and editing or book indexing by reading books recommended by the professional associations for medical and science writers, biology editors, or back-of-book indexers.

So far, there is no such thing as a certified medical editor, indexer, abstractor, publicist, ad copywriter, video scriptwriter, or print writer. However, many courses and continuing education materials are always available from the trade and professional writers' and editors' associations. Many courses are offered at conventions for continuing education for medical writers and editors.

Attend Medical Meetings and Press Conferences

Medical professional research institutes, groups, and associations often invite the press to attend medical meetings to mingle with and interview physicians and scientists on their latest research. Attend these meetings with other journalists and freelancers, physicians, and scientists.

Attend the conventions and visit the monthly or quarterly meetings of your local chapters of some of these organizations.

Open an On-Line Medical Editing Service

Open an on-line medical editing service, using your computer and taped interviews to produce biomedical, scientific, and technical manuscripts. Also, you may specialize in health information reporting for the health and fitness or nutrition mass media publications.

Biomedical Curriculum Writing and Editing

Curriculum design writing is a burgeoning, big industry. Write or edit training and curriculum materials for careers in medical insurance billing, transcription, medical editing, or science journalism. Write about, report on, or edit training materials in medical records technology training. Some examples are writing about indexing and coding training materials and curriculum design books or trade journals (magazines of the industry).

Write about or edit materials that help to train others to eventually become accredited records technicians or registered records administrators by writing books about the subject without actually being one. Medical communications includes reporting and interviewing skills, courseware design writing, instructional technology, distance teaching materials publishing, and health sciences editing.

Freelancing For the Medical and Science Market

As an independent contractor, even if you don't have a degree, you can work at home freelance as a medical editor, journalist, or indexer in your own business. You can be a success story case history manager and interview people by telephone about why they switched from one medical product to another. Critique other science writers' materials and edit it for practice in writing according to the guidelines of the particular publication.

Start freelancing by attending conventions and writing summaries of what medical papers were presented. You can abstract or summarize medical articles from journals for abstracting services. They're listed in your Yellow Pages phone directory and in directories of abstracting services that you can research in public or university libraries.

You can find dozens of markets for your freelance writing in the medical field. Freelance writers interested in medical or scientific subjects are sometimes asked to contribute articles to encyclopedias designed for high-school students.

Associate Editors Are Also Needed

Starting out with the job title of associate editor can get you started in your medical communications career as a language specialist. Associate editors also are hired to work in other countries for chemical or medical news published by professional societies, such as the American Chemical Society, or other scientific and professional groups.

Apply For Open Forums, Seminars, Scholarships, and Grants for Science Journalists and Freelance Writers

The American Chemical Society offers science reporter's workshops, an open forum for science writers seeking to expand their skill and knowledge in science writing. Twenty applicants a year are selected, for example, to participate in this particular workshop. You can apply for science writing fellowships at a variety of labs, such as the Marine Biological Laboratory in Woods Hole, MA. The American Cancer Society offers a science writer's seminar.

Work is sometimes available as a public information representative or grant proposal writer for a variety of universities. Go down to your local grants funding office focusing on medical funding and go through their books and guidelines on how to write medical grant proposals. Courses are also offered through extended studies departments of colleges on grant proposal writing for medical and non-profit organizations.

Apply for fellowships for writers, journalists, and freelancers. There are fellowships offered, such as the Sigma-Tau Foundation's Alzheimer Journalism Fellowship for stories written or broadcast about the medical, scientific, or psychological aspect of Alzheimer's disease.

Look For A Niche, Seek Out Alternative Pathways

There are many alternatives and possibilities for advancing your career in the direction of biomedical communications or medical news writing and editorial work.

For example, medical journalists have written books on subjects ranging from agoraphobia to how to identify and reduce your risks for a variety of diseases.

Look at the monthly list of books written by journalist members of the National Association of Science Writers. Many are freelance writers working at home in biomedical communications, writing, or on-line editing. There's even a specialty in television and radio medical news broadcasting/reporting for persons whose aptitudes are more oral than print journalism and book publishing-oriented.

An updated national directory of university science communications courses and scholarships is published by the University of Wisconsin-Madison, School of Journalism. For further information, write to Sharon Dunwoody, School of Journalism and Mass Communication, University of Wisconsin, 821 University Avenue, Madison, WI 53706.

To educate yourself, go to annual science writers' meetings held by the American Heart Association, the American Cancer Association, and the AMA. These meetings last a few days. Other medical associations hold day-long seminars.

I learned more about medical writing by attending week-long medical meetings and one-day seminars for journalists than I ever did in my graduate writing course work in college. You can even write to schools of public health to find out what kind of meetings or fellowships are open to biomedical communicators and journalists or freelancers.

Numerous medical reporters lack science degrees. They could be liberal arts or journalism school graduates or nurses and therapists seeking writing careers. We learn by going to medical meetings, reading, and interviewing.

If you're a transcriber now, don't ever be frightened away by the fact that you didn't major in biology. You can learn and write at the same time and check all facts with the experts like you do when transcribing unfamiliar medical dictation.

There are plenty of books and journal articles in medical and university libraries to re-read. Practice making the complex clearer to understand for mass media readers or for your technical audience. (I once had a job as a technical writer rewriting computer manuals. I had to shorten sentences to ten words each and make the long words easier to understand.)

You can become a health reporter. Don't try to cover all sides. Medical writing is a challenge to reporters and editors with liberal arts backgrounds or with a transcription background and no degree.

Never let your training or lacks of it bias you. Your job is to interview the experts and check back with them to make sure they mean what you say in print. Keep your interviews on tape so you don't misquote. The first rule you learn is to never take a press release at face value.

Most of the work you'll do may be as a writer of articles who will gather background for lay-language newsletters and other publications covering a medical institution's advance in treatment and prevention or research and education.

You'll use your terminology and knowledge of anatomy and pathophysiology in ways similar to the person with a B.A. in biology who tries to get a journalism job in the public affairs office. What you'll use is your transcription skills now transferred to the job of "paying attention to detail and institutional information."

Advancement is to publications project manager or director of public relations, marketing communications, or publications. You may start out as an editorial assistant if you're organized and good at proofreading and fact checking publications.

The medical editorial assistant provides support for an editorial staff. For this job, you'll need an interest in biomedicine and some editorial office experience (journalism workshop course or public relations/public affairs volunteer experience or internship).

To create an internship, call the public affairs department of a biomedical organization and ask for unpaid internships on a part-time basis to gain experience. Tell them that you're using your medical transcription skills in an expanded environment. You'll be hired when you present yourself as the least financial risk to a new employer. With medical writing, editing, and indexing skills, you will advance vertically up the career ladder instead of only horizontally.

Biomedical Communications as a Career Stepping Stone to Publications Management

You'll work on written reports, attend conferences, and interview people as you check facts. You won't be typing constantly, and your wrists will get a well deserved rest. Biomedical communications is one field where you can work as a freelancer and not have your advanced age, production quota per typed line, or keyboarding speed discussed or electronically monitored.

Freelancing For the Federal Government

Freelance work also exists with the government, for example, with the National Institutes of Health, and other DC agencies, national public radio, Time-Life Books, Science magazine, etc. Target institutes where they need your interest in special knowledge.

With the recommended reading below, you can begin to prepare yourself at home to become a medical editor or writer if you're already a medical transcriber or student of transcription.

Teaching Yourself Publications Management, Editing, and Writing

It's possible to learn medical copyediting and proofreading by yourself. Start out by learning basic copyediting and practicing on medical manuscripts using your knowledge of terminology. Then proceed to study medical journalism.

Volunteer your writing services to medical professional association's publications and trade journals. Call the trade journals for the allied health fields and ask to be a stringer (freelancer on call). Interview professionals by phone and transcribe what they said, editing the material into a brief article jam-packed with facts and tips.

Correspondence courses are offered at the USDA Graduate School in Washington, DC. (You don't need an undergraduate degree to take these courses at home for college credit.) The USDA Graduate School offers a certificate in professional editing and writing, including several courses in medical and technical editing, writing, indexing, and managing the editing processes and department. Write to them at 600 Maryland Ave. SW, Washington, DC, Washington, DC.

Read basic books on technical writing and how to eliminate excessive wordiness in medical publications. These books are available from the Society for Technical Communication or the American Association for Medical Writing and National Association of Science Writers, Inc. A few basic starters' books are recommended below.

Medical English Usage and Abusage, Edith Schwager
Oryx Press, Phoenix, AZ 1991

Copyediting, a practical guide, Karen Judd
Crisp Publications, Inc., 990
95 First St.
Los Altos, CA 94022

Style, J.M. Williams
HarperCollins Publishers, 1989

Technical Writing (second edition)
Paul V. Anderson
Harcourt Brace Jovanovich, 1989
8th floor
Orlando, Florida 32887

• Note: Find a copy of "Uniform Requirements for Manuscripts Submitted to Biomedical Journals" (and supplemental statements from the International Committee of Medical Journal Editors.) Write to the American College of Physicians, Independence Mall West, Sixth Street, Race, Philadelphia, PA 19106-1572.

In addition to books and learning materials, professional and trade associations may be of help offering instruction, continuing education, volunteer opportunities, internships or a chance to work on a newsletter or help set up speakers' panels at conventions. Ask how you may be of service and learn from your experience. Then share meaning with others and communicate. For further information write to the following trade and professional associations that are very helpful for writers in the fields of medicine or science:

American Medical Writers Association
40 West Gude Drive, Suite 101
Rockville, MD 20850-1192
http://www.amwa.org/default.asp?ID=1

National Association of
Science Writers, Inc.
P.O. Box 890, Hedgesville, WV 25427
http://www.nasw.org/

American Society of Journalists and Authors
1501 Broadway, Suite 302
New York, NY 10036
http://www.asja.org

Society for Technical Communication
http://www.stc.org/

Association of Professional Writing Consultants
http://www.consultingsuccess.org/index.htm

Council of the Advancement of Science Writing
P.O. Box 910
Hedgesville, WV 25427

http://www.casw.org/
Careers in Science Writing: http://www.casw.org/careers.htm

World Association of Medical Editors
http://www.wame.org/
http://www.wame.org/index.htm

Text and Academic Authors Association
TAA
P.O. Box 76477
St. Petersburg, FL
http://www.taaonline.net/

Education Writers Association
2122 P Street, NW Suite 201
Washington, DC 20037
http://www.ewa.org/

Council of Biology Editors
http://www.monroecc.edu/depts/library/cbe.htm

American Society of Indexers (for indexing careers)
10200 West 44th Avenue, Suite 304,
Wheat Ridge, CO 80033
http://www.asindexing.org/site/index.html

Society of Professional Journalists
Eugene S. Pulliam National Journalism Center,
3909 N. Meridian St., Indianapolis, IN 46208
http://www.spj.org/

2

Samples of Published Medical Writing

Here are some of my published medical writing samples for a general consumer audience. Note the style of language and the emphasis on not using medical terminology. Even if you're a medical language specialist, the general reader wants everything explained clearly in plain language. If you have to use a scientific or medical term, define it for the reader without distracting from the topic.

We'll start with a review of my published article that had been archived on the Web at HEALTHNET NEWS VOL. XI, NO. 4, WINTER 1995, Lyman Maynard Stowe Library

University of Connecticut Health Center. The Web site where the review of my article is located is at: http://library.uchc.edu/departm/hnet/winter95.html. Below you can see the archived review.

"**Anne Hart**, a medical journalist, was unhappy with her doctor's response to her questions regarding different treatment methods for the symptoms of menopause. She decided to do her own research to find answers to her questions. She was interested in finding information about natural yam-derived progesterone as an alternative to hormone replacement therapy (HRT). Hart believed the estrogen in HRT was the cause of her dangerously high blood pressure. Using the Internet to access newsgroups and WWW sites, she not only found information on alternative therapies but also physicians who were able to answer her questions about these treatments. She later successfully investigated a medical problem for her husband.

In this very informative article, Hart describes her journey on the Internet. She offers tips on how to successfully search for a wide range of health information and gives her "picks" for the best WWW sites and newsgroups. (Reviewed by Tate A.) Second opinion. **Internet World** 1996 February : 42-44, 46, 48."

MENOPAUSE AND BEYOND ALTERNATIVE RESOURCES AND INFORMATION ONLINE

Alternative Resources Online for Menopause and Beyond

Through the Internet, you can obtain information your doctor hasn't got time to give you, and talk to people who share your problems.

By Anne Hart

I have found that doctors don't always have the time or breadth of knowledge to discuss alternative, customized solutions to my family's healthcare needs. That's why I turned to the Internet. After searching the Net for Web sites, support groups, or little-known health newsletters, I found dozens of physicians who offered to give me answers to my specific questions via e-mail.

Each member of my family required a different healthcare service and support group to address their particular problems. In my case, I am allergic to synthetic progestin, which eases the side effects of menopause. At the health-maintenance organization (HMO) to which I am a member, I asked my doctor for natural, yam-derived progesterone. He refused to prescribe it because he said it wasn't yet approved by the FDA, which left me with no alternatives to prevent osteoporosis, for which I'm at high risk. Instead I was put on hormone-replacement therapy, which involves taking oral estrogen. I believed that the oral estrogen was raising my blood pressure sky high. When I mentioned this to my doctor's nurse, she snapped, "Prove it."

So I set off on my journey to prove it. First I checked the **alt.support.menopause** newsgroup, which was extremely helpful. I posted the following question: *Is anyone else using a high soy and vegetarian diet, the herb black cohosh, and natural, yam-derived, progesterone cream for menopause—to help prevent bone loss—instead of the usual estrogen and progestin? If so, what are your comments and experiences?*

The replies were practical, useful, and factual, providing medical references, titles of medical journal articles, and book bibliographies, as well as personal experiences and encouragement. For example, one person pointed me to an article entitled "Risks of Estrogens and Progestogens" in the December 1990 issue of

Maturitas, an English-language European medical journal. The author, Dr. Marc L'Hermite, found that five to seven percent of women on conjugated equine estrogens could get severe high blood pressure and that they would return to normal when the hormone-replacement therapy was withdrawn. A bibliographic reference to this article also appeared in Dr. Lonnie Barbach's book *The Pause*. Not one physician at my HMO had mentioned these concerns.

To obtain more information about what alternative health solutions were available and how particular products would change my body or health, I searched the Web under the keywords "menopause," "alternative healthcare," "herbs," "homeopathy," and "naturopathy." I also looked under "natural progesterone."

Through this search I found the *MenoTimes*, a quarterly journal published in San Rafael, Calif. I subscribed because it had the information I sought on Dr. John Lee's book *Natural Progesterone: The Multiple Roles of a Remarkable Hormone*.

Also through my search I found a laboratory that would test my saliva and tell me whether my hormones were balanced. Most of all, I wanted to know how taking natural progesterone would affect my fast thyroid and adrenaline-drenched body, with its low blood sugar and excess insulin production. My HMO physicians did not answer these questions, but told me that going off conjugated equine estrogen and synthetic progestin was like a diabetic going off insulin. On the Net I found physicians who answered my letters, labs that sold natural progesterone cream that I could use to prevent bone loss after menopause, and other labs that could monitor my condition until I found a doctor in my community who would listen to alternative solutions to menopausal questions.

I even found the Menopause Matters page created by Susan Czernicka, who said she "learned about herbal treatment of menopause when there were too few resources available to help her with her many symptoms and too few medical providers with open minds." She will answer questions sent to her at susan270@world.std.com.

For those who don't have Web access, there is the Menopause mailing list. To subscribe, send e-mail to listserv@ psuhmc.hmc.psu.edu with **subscribe menopaus *Your Name*** in the message body.

The "black cohosh" that I mentioned in my letter to the **alt.support.menopause** newsgroup is an estrogenic herb and vasodilator, and I wanted to find out how safe it was and whether it was as good for menopause as the homeopaths and naturopaths claimed, as well as how much to use and what effects it would have. I found the **alt. folklore.herbs** newsgroup helpful, as well as articles by Anthony Brook entitled "Why Herbs?" and "Historic Uses of Herbs" at the <u>Drum Holistic Herbs</u> page.

I wanted to find out everything I could about natural progesterone, so I went to the Health and Science page at <u>Polaris Network</u>, which described itself as "A Guide to Understanding and Controlling PMS, Fertility, Menopause, and Osteoporosis." It contained information about natural progesterone and how it balances the side effects of unopposed estrogen, how it's required for proper thyroid function and progestin counterparts in the drug industry. It also offered a seemingly sound scientific and unbiased evaluation of how certain hormones affect the system, what the hormone's results are on various bodily functions, and side effects. And it had an excellent bibliography of books and medical journal articles on osteoporosis reversal using natural progesterone.

I wanted to query a physician about the high blood pressure resulting from the equine oral estrogen I was taking, and at the <u>Atlanta Reproductive Health Centre</u> page I was able to send e-mail to a doctor who answered my question quickly, providing information that I could consider when making my final decisions or in looking further. His answer was more to the point than the counseling I had received from my own physician.

Another doctor of mine had wanted to give me high blood pressure medicine on top of the estrogen and synthetic progestin. I asked him to consider the alternative—taking me off the hormones to see whether a low-salt diet and exercise could change things—because before I went on hormones my blood pressure wasn't high.

The Internet became one of my best alternative healthcare information resources after the last of three reproductive endocrinologists I saw (not affiliated with my HMO) told me to wait two months to see how I felt off the hormones.
Menopause is a mega-business. More than 100 books a year fill the store shelves on this subject and more than 3,500 baby boomers enter menopause daily. This captivated audience represents a huge market for makers of hormones, vitamins,

and other specialty products, much of which is advertised on the Web. So a wealth of information has appeared on the Internet to meet the needs of the 38- to 55-year-olds undergoing menopause, as well as younger women with PMS, infertility, and contraception concerns.

Another resource I found informative was the Women's Health Hot Line news-letter. Its topics include infertility, endometriosis, contraception, sexually trans-mitted diseases, stress, menopause, and PMS. Most of all, it doesn't close its pages to alternative therapies for women who can't tolerate standard hormone replacement therapy.

Hernia Hunt

This year my husband needed hernia repair surgery, but his busy HMO surgeon spent only a very short time briefing him a month before his surgery. Because it would take hours to describe in detail what is done during hernia repair surgery, he searched on the topic using Web search engines, which yielded a list of infor-mation about all kinds of hernias. The most thorough site discovered was the Hernia Information Home Page in England. It included articles that explained such things as the benefits of using mesh rather than stitches to close incisions. Information about hiatal hernias and diaphragmatic hernias could be found at the Collaborative Hypertext of Radiology. There was more information about hernias on the Net than my husband could possibly find time to read.

After seeing shark cartilage in many health food stores, my husband asked his sur-geon about its ability to aid in faster wound-healing. The surgeon laughed, yet I found several references to articles discussing shark cartilage on the Internet. Some medical journal articles on the healing and other properties and uses of shark cartilage can be found on the Simone Protective Pharmaceuticals page. Also at the site I found health-style questionnaires, in-depth descriptions of a variety of nutrient products, and how each product affects the body. You'll also find information about where to order or buy shark cartilage from pharmacists.

Search Tips

From the many healthcare sites I visited, my three-ring binder is packed with more than 500 pages of answers to questions. Productive keyword searches can be made using terms such as "alternative health," "healthcare," "medical," "medi-cine," "nurses," "nutrition," "pharmacy," "physicians," and "smart drugs." I found the search word "healthcare" to be more specific for asking personal medical questions than trying to search under the word "health."

Some sites are best reached through links on dedicated healthcare Web pages. For example, Subhas Roy has a created a page with links to 25 other Internet health sites at <u>Health Info</u>. There also is a large collection of links at the <u>Internet Medical and Mental Health Resources</u> page. It's maintained by Jeanine Wade, Ph.D., a licensed psychologist in Austin, Texas. One particularly comprehensive directory of health and medical sites on the Web is <u>MedWeb</u>, which lists Web sites and mailing lists in 70 categories, from AIDS to toxicology.

One of the best medical referral Web sites I found was <u>Richard C. Bowyer's</u> page. (You'll find it when you scroll past all his genealogy information.) Bowyer's page has links to numerous sites, such as U.S. hospitals, medical resources, medical journals, medical schools, medical students, medicolegal resources, oncology, pathology, and different surgical disciplines, such as plastic surgery, general surgery, laparoscopic surgery, and telesurgery. Healthcare workers of all specializations also can find job opportunities on some of these sites.

My son, who recently became a physician, was interested in <u>Medline</u>, a collection of medical and scientific reports used by physicians, articles on the educational needs of physicians and the public, physicians' supplies, prescriptions, and advice by pharmacists about drugs. Clinical cancer information that is intended for physicians is useful to patients as well. There is a listing of surgeons according to the types of surgery they perform, the notes of the Physician Reliance Network, and a Gopher menu of physicians listed according to their specialty.

As for informative newsletters available on the Net, I highly recommend the <u>University of California at Berkeley Wellness Letter at the Electronic Newsstand</u>. It contains the latest news of preventive medicine and practical advice—including information on nutrition, weight control, self-care, prevention of cancer and heart disease, exercise, and dental care.

As a medical journalist, I found the <u>Journal of the American Medical Association</u> (JAMA) to be a reliable resource.

If you are looking for a description of a particular drug, the <u>Physician's GenRx</u> Web site provides a database of drugs you can search. You must register first.

In seeking answers to my health questions, I found the Internet to be a valuable source for a wide range of healthcare information. I'm sure your efforts will be rewarded, too.

Selected Health Sites

Anesthesiology & Surgery Center *Offers travel warnings and immunization, medical dictionary.*

Cancer Related Links *Facts, figures, prevention.*

Harvard Medical Gopher *Harvard publications, access to the Countway Library's online catalog (HOLLIS), and medicine.*

Health Letter on the CDC

Health on the Internet Newsletter *Links to NewsPages, CNN Food & Health, MEDwire, describes new health-related Web sites, topic of the month.*

HyperDOC *Sponsored by the National Library of Medicine.*

LifeNet *Positive thinking and right-to-life point of views. Discussion about euthanasia.*

The Mayo Clinic *tour of the Mayo clinic; description of programs.*

Med Help International *Provides medical information about many illnesses. Treatment is described in layman's terms.*

Mednews *A biweekly newsletter that welcomes submissions.*

Medical Information Resource Center *Lists and a referral directory.*

Medicine OnLine *Career-related educational content and discussion groups.*

Medscape *For health professionals and consumers. Bulletin boards and a quiz testing your knowledge of surgery. Registration required.*

The National Organization of Physicians Who Care *Nonprofit organization ensuring quality healthcare. Newsletters, articles about Medicare reform and HMOs.*

OncoLink, the University of Pennsylvania Cancer Resource *Thorough information about pediatric and adult cancers.*

Physicians Guide to the Internet *For new physicians.*

Robert Wood Johnson Foundation Gopher *Biological archives at Indiana university, molecular biology database, NYU Medical Gopher.*

◆   ◆   ◆

During the 1970s, writing under my pen names or maiden name, I sold most of my health, medical, and nutrition articles to business magazines such as Registered Representative, which published most of my healthcare articles during the last seventies and/or early 1980s. The articles below represent my emphasis on writing about the health and nutrition issues particularly for the type of reader of the particular magazine. In these cases, the magazines were directed at stock brokers, called registered representatives. Thus, I emphasized writing medical and health or fitness articles for Registered Representative, a magazine that is distributed nationally primarily to stock brokers.

The articles written were based on telephone interviews with a variety of stockbrokers during the early 1980s. If you write medical articles, as a writer who presumably has no science background, your best bet is to target magazines in other than medical areas such as business publications. Contact publications that might be interested in articles on fitness for their particular readers who might be business persons, stock brokers, teachers, therapists, chefs, soldiers, parents, or office workers.

INNER CLOCKS

Timing the Monday slumps and the Thursday jumps

By Anne Hart

There is no aspect of human biology that is not influenced by our daily internal clock rhythms. This, in turn, influences the way in which we conduct our daily business.

Our blood pressure rises between 8:00 A.M. and 12 Noon, and then starts dropping until its midnight low. There's an internal clock governing our hormone levels and our heartbeat, all following different clocks that may bear only a slight relation to our daily cycle.

The best predictor of job performance is body temperature. As it falls from a 10 p.m. zenith of 99 degrees to a pre-dawn nadir of 97 degrees, our mental functions drop. We perform best when all the body's clocks are in sync. When our mechanisms fall out of step, we make errors or have accidents.

Memory peaks at 11 a.m., but math skills drop off at noon. Business performance levels fall just after lunch. By late afternoon, stress can be handled more effectively.

The internal clock is as individual as a fingerprint. What is certain is that the person you are in the morning is different from the one you are at night.

Once you have determined what your high and low energy levels are, you will be better able to adjust your prospecting and selling activities to more efficient and profitable time slots.

Each morning Joan, a 32-year old stockbroker, rises at 4:30 a.m., rushes her three preschoolers to the babysitter, jogs around the beach and reaches her office with most other West Coast RR's, at 6:00 a.m. She is responsible for servicing a hefty client book, learning new product information, cold calling, and processing her own paper work.

As a single parent, after Joan puts in a full day, she picks up her children and arrives home to a full evening of unshared housework. She grosses as high as the top RR's in her firm. How does she get her second wind?

Joan has tuned into her internal clock to tell her why she thinks and works better on some days than on others. Biorhythm/internal clock theory is medically called chronobiology. (The difference between biorhythms and internal clocks is that biorhythms measure the physical, emotional and intellectual cycles, while internal clocks measure mood, memory and body temperature during a 24-hour cycle.) It supposes that each person has a built-in biological clock that regulates the levels of various hormones and the rates or chemical processes in response to internal and environmental cues.

Individuals respond to this regulation by periodic changes in their growth and behavior patterns. Jet lag is one example of what happens when the internal clock is out of whack.

Back in the early 1980s, in order to interview a biorhythms expert for this article, I spoke to special chronobiological consultant, Ralph Zuranski (in the early 1980s) whose business it is (at the time of the interview) to teach salespersons and executives how to structure their business to keep in harmony with their internal clock so that maximum productivity can be achieved.

To write this article for Registered Representative magazine, I talked to numerous stockbrokers, called Registered Representatives. When you interview people for a health-oriented article to be published in a business emphasis magazine, make sure you have plenty of quotes both from the experts in the health field and from people in a business related to the magazine's audience.

I've taken out the last names of the stock brokers that I interviewed and the names of their companies, since the article appeared in print more than 25 years ago. What I wanted to emphasize is that I spoke to both a chronological consultant and the people employed in a field related to the business magazine publishing my articles.

When you write your own articles or books, talk to experts and people who use or have an interest in the topic you emphasize. Quotes from the experts and the users of healthcare products, systems, or services are necessary to lend credibility and references to your work so readers can do fact-checking or contact the experts who may have a service to offer.

You can blend this type of medical writing with corporate success stories and case histories. If you use success stories, emphasize results and problems solved. Your article should contain step-by-step instructions reader can follow to solve similar problems or achieve results. Note in the article, I mentioned what the expert determines or achieves—as in the sample below.

Zuranski can determine when salespeople will have a "critical" day, and how to use the internal clock to their best advantage. Zuranski evaluates the performance level of the sales executive on a scale according to their biorhythms. When Zuranksi applied this evaluation to the performance level of the San Diego Chargers in 1989, he found two types of players.

One type performed at an average level all the time, while the other type manifested extreme activity whether that type played a fantastic game or a terrible one. With the stockbrokers (also known in their occupation as Registered Representatives or RRs) interviewed, the same pattern was revealed. Some had a peak activity period between 7:00 a.m. and 11:00 a.m., whereas others showed no energy high points or valley of fatigue at any special hour of the workday.

To examine the internal clocks, Zuranski did a compatibility study between executives (or players) and the manager (or coach), the assistant coach, and all the trainers and persons working with the athletes (or RR's). The compatibility study between the trainers and the coaches was vital in order that all could be aware of the similarity of the energy flow between them. For each game he predicted on a scale of 4 to 10 at what level he thought each member or the team would play. He always gave his prediction to the coaches before the game, and they, in turn, used the prediction to evaluate their athletes.

With RR's, Zuranski uses computer producing biorhythms charts to obtain a workup on each RR. "I sit down with them," he said, "and ask how they felt that day. This is to see if I can pinpoint on the chart if there is a correlation and which cycle has the most influence."

When the correlation is determined where the person feels most high or low the results are put in a diary.

"We keep a record of their productivity growth," Zuranski added, "to see how much they were selling that day. "We keep track of their production level for at least a month. That way we can look back at their cycle to determine when they perform their best. If they don't perform, their cash gross is a good indicating factor or a low day."

"We take the cash gross of a salesperson and evaluate it according to what their biological cycles were on that lucky day. All three bio-rhythms go into their output (mood, memory and body temperature). This corresponds to the physical, emotional and intellectual cycle. If all three rhythms were going into the output, Zuranski assigns that RR a larger quota of work because that person has more energy going in one direction.

According to Dennis, a Registered Representative, biorhythms have been helpful to him. "I used to study biorhythms back when I taught school in 1965," Dennis said.

"On a number of occasions, when, things were really bad, I would check the chart to see where I was. When I was emotionally down that day, my biorhythms chart showed I was either in a down pattern or near the bottom of the trough. More often than not, the cycles were indicative of how I was performing."

The only times Dennis checked his biorhythm chart was when he was emotionally stressed. "Physically, I was not at a high. If I checked any chart, my emotional cycle would probably be high and my physical cycle would probably be down. My guess us that if I looked at my chart, I would have found it to read the way I felt."

Dennis illustrated how he used his biorhythm computer, a small hand calculator. "You take your biorhythm calculator and kick in your birth date, plus the current date, and it comes out with a number for each of the three areas that measure your physical, intellectual, and emotional highs and lows. These areas correlate to the medical findings that daily circadian rhythms occur in mood, memory and body temperature within our body clocks."

Dennis found that at 7:00 a.m. he starts to get geared up. By 10:00 a.m. he's consistently at his best. Around 11:00 a.m. he starts to tail off at a continually accelerating degree.

"By noon," he says, "I feel fatigued, but it's usually because I've done so much in the first three or four hours."

Zuranski would want to find out if Dennis was feeling fatigued on the day of the week that was the same as Dennis' birth date.

"I would determine whether Dennis was born on a day numbered during the week," Zuranski says, "because that's the time each week that any person would want to be most aware and most balanced. For example, if Dennis was born on Nov. 18th and this was July 18th, he would be especially receptive and sensitive to his cycle on that day of the week."

Dennis continued, "I start getting excited about the market at 12:15; I've been a broker for 10 years, and it seems that the market goes up or down between 12:10 and 1:40, changing again during the last 15 minutes."

When the market goes down, Dennis feels stressed more easily, as do most other RR's interviewed. He feels most RR's are bullish by nature and adds, "I don't eat breakfast or lunch. I leave work at 2:00."

After work Dennis has what he terms his "success-hour", during which time he gets physical exercise by running.

At work his success hour is when he writes a big ticket. He notices his highest peak of elation when the market closes.

Another RR who firmly believes in and frequently checks biorhythms and internal clock cycles to predict work performance is Rachel, a Registered Representative. When she travels, Rachel checks her biorhythm chart.

"On the day I had to go back to New York to take my exam," she says, "I had two cross-over days, so I immediately knew it would it be a terrible day. And it was.

"Although I was well prepared, I flunked my exam. I charted my biorhythms about a week before I took the test, and learned that the exam day was on one of my critical days.

"During the exam, it was like I really wasn't there."

"The next working day I took another exam along with the other people who failed the test and received a 90 on it. Nothing changed. I was just as well prepared to take the exam as on the previous day, yet that first day I knew I was going to flunk the test as soon as I walked into the room."

If Rachel is going to have an important appointment with a client especially one concerning a substantial amount of money, she checks her biorhythms to see whether it's a good day for her to be the most effective.

"If it's not a good day," she admitted, "I set up a joint appointment with someone else." For Rachel, biorhythms are used more to avoid the negative than to accentuate the positive.

"I don't have any special second winds" Rachel explained. "My peak is at noon and from there on, I start to wind down throughout the day. Business pours in heavily between 9: 00 and 11:00 a.m., and I find the most enjoyable part of the working day is 2:00 to 4:00 p.m."

Gina, a Registered Representative, bought a dog to wake her up at 5:00 a.m. for her morning jog. Eventually, she switched to a 1:00 p. m. aerobics class. Rated on a scale of 1 to 10, she said she is at 5 when she first walks into work. Her lowest point occurs at 3:00 p.m., and then she gets her second wind by 4:00.

She explained, "From 4:00 to 6:00 p.m. I'm very productive, because there's no one in the office."

Most Registered Representatives interviewed stated that they enjoyed prospecting from an office after hours or from their homes in the evening because they had the most control and least distraction in their environment. For some, it was pointed out as the most point in their workday. Physical activity during working hours was common.

Gina doesn't jog as much now, because she saunas every Tuesday and Thursday, while the rest of the week she is busy with her aerobics class. For Gina the late afternoon, between 4:00 and 6:00 p.m., is the least stressful time of the day to handle an irate client. Gina cold-calls clients from 9:00 to 5:00 PM.

Gloria, a Registered Representative, also exercises during the day. Like most of the RR's interviewed, Gloria is a morning person. She finds release from stress in walking along the beach, a few blocks from her office.

Informally, Gloria has monitored her work performance in accordance with the time of day, and structured her work to keep in tune with her internal clock. She explained, "I function best while drumming up sales between 8:00 a.m. and 1:00 p.m. That first hour, is I'm hitting my peak production.

"Since in the afternoon there's no second wind—I'm going downhill by then, I begin prospecting. To relieve stress, I take hardy walks along the oceanside. Indoors, to relieve the stress that begins in my shoulders, I sit back and relax at my desk. Business is structured to coincide with my high energy level in the morning."

Morning people have a higher body temperature than the afternoon or evening person. That's what gives them that early morning burst of energy. However, not every Registered Representative is a morning person, as Maurice, another Registered Representative, is quick to admit. "By nature I'm not a morning person, but after twenty years on the job, my system has adjusted to putting out its peak performance in the morning.

"I suffer from Monday syndrome. On Mondays I seem to be at my lowest level. I notice a pickup on Tuesday and Wednesday, and by Thursday, I'm keenest. On Friday I begin to wind down."

Maurice notices that most of the Registered Representatives in his office are aware of the Monday slump and the Thursday jump—a high point of productivity. "Inevitably," Maurice says, "my system is low on Monday and so is business. It is a pattern."

John, another Registered Representative at a different firm, uses the earliest morning hours to his best advantage. Consequently, morning hours are when his peak production level occurs.

"After lunch, around 1:30 p.m.," John said, "I become more articulate and motivated when many Registered Representatives are going into their slump fatigue of the afternoon, that's when I get my second wind and do most of my prospecting. That's between 3:00 and 4:00 p.m.

"It's a most refreshing experience. I find that when clients are winding down in the late afternoon, they are most accessible to business.

"I put myself in time locks," John continued. "I have certain goal time frames that may last three hours each. Accordingly, I do my cold calling between 9:00 a.m. and noon. Another time lock is reserved for paperwork, while in the evening I organize my plan for the next day by writing down a list of things to do.

"If too many things are going on at once, I put all of them in time frames. During stressful moments it helps to put things in perspective, to sit down and paint a picture of why I'm under stress."

John feels that 10:00 a.m. is the most "socially acceptable" part of the day, a time when working people are in their peak production period and enjoying their best mood of the day.

Rachel Paulin agrees that ten in the morning is the best time of day most experience their best "internal clock" mood of the day.

Dennis concurs. "I'm consistently at my best at 10:00 a.m."

Gina added that, "My memory is at its peak between 10:00 and 11:00 a.m. That's when I'm really cooking and have all the inputs of the day. I know what all the numbers are doing. I feel comfortable with the market, and have a handle on what I'm selling. All in all, it's a very safe feeling time for me."

3

What to Emphasize In Medical Writing for General Consumer Publications

In the previous chapter, you learned that medical writing for general consumer or business publications emphasizes making the complex and technical easy to understand and clear. If you're writing about biorhythms, you need to explain to readers that they are inner clocks.

Focus on what the objectives or goals are of tracking your inner clocks. As a medical writer for non-medical publications, you need to explain that the purpose of writing about inner clocks is to tell the reader in a nutshell that there is a time, a circadian inner clock and rhythm which is different for each individual.

Your inner clock tells you when memory peaks, when math skills drop off, and when you're most likely to pass an exam. Medical writing for general magazines is meant to show readers where they can turn when their job is making them or their employees sick. What's the purpose of medical writing for general consumer magazines? It's about how to make your job your friend or how to feel better doing what's good for your system.

In science writing for non-scientific or business magazines, the simple explanation works. Don't talk down to readers, but explain anything technical, assuming the reader can be a professional in another field, a stay-at-home parent, or someone from any occupation or lifestyle who wants clearly explained information without confusion.

Keep medical articles about 1,000 words in length. The magazine you've queried with a letter to get an assignment usually will give you a specific length—usually 1,200-1,600 words. Some publications have space for only 800 words. Newspapers may only want a 400-word column. Some publications will have space for up to 2,000 words. However, it's easier to sell a health-oriented article that's about 1,000 words.

Here's a sample below of a medical article that was snapped up by Registered Representative in the early 1980s. The article is about stress reduction. To slant the article to the magazine for stockbrokers, I interviewed stockbrokers (Registered Representatives). For privacy, I've removed the last name and name of the company that the person worked for, since the article appeared more than 25 years ago.

There were titles and subtitles on the article. Note the main title is "Making Your Job Your Friend." This article could also work for a magazine for older adults, for a parenting magazine or for a magazine on marriage and relationships. It would work for an inspirational, health-oriented, or fitness magazine as well as for business publications.

The main point of this article is that your stressor may be the race against time or your job could become your personal battle. These types of health-oriented articles are ageless and don't go out of date because they emphasize unchanging values—making your job your friend.

Peruse the published writing sample below. Note it does not go out of date. This article could have been published today or a generation ago and would still be marketable to business, self-help, and general consumer magazines. It's about making your job your friend. The article illustrates the effects of stress that could occur when you are married to your job. The facts and examples represent universal concepts.

Medical writing is salable to non-medical publications when the writing emphasizes solutions to problems and situations that everyone experiences. That's why articles emphasizing simple, effective solutions to the notion of marrying your job or making your job your friend are nourishment. And nourishment, like commitment, sells to general consumer, business, inspirational, and educational magazines.

Making Your Job Your Friend
In Sickness And In Health: When You Marry Your Job

At the age of 70, Bill is the type of guy you would think was immune to occupational stress sickness. He has been a hard-driving, tough-to-please-in-making-employee-evaluations supervisor since 1946 and still puts in nine-hour workdays. Fisher walks two miles to work each day, goes mountain climbing and backpacking, and occasionally jogs. He stays away from fatty foods, smoking, and worry. Three years ago doctors gave him only two weeks to live.

"Work was my enemy, but the battle for money was my number one goal," he said. "The need to win struggled mercilessly against my fear of losing."

Fisher's body became so run down he couldn't comfortably walk around the block. Fisher had put everything into that second job and had borrowed money to relocate.

He Was Married To His Job

Long before Fisher started his present job, the previous business he worked for went bankrupt. One year after joining his next company and moving all of his clients with him, he received a call telling him that his new outfit also would be closing down within two weeks.

"I went home," he said, "and had my first in a series of severe heart attacks, ending in bypass surgery." Yet within three years, Fisher earned every dollar back for each of his clients. Today he's in a job where he has stopped struggling against time and work. He advised, "Don't take your job tasks as your personal battle. There's not plenty of time to play later when you've made your money or earned your pension. Your body is not invincible.

"As you make more money or gain more promotions, or become a supervisor or manager after climbing up the ranks, your lifestyle costs more to maintain," Fisher confessed. "Learning to protect my employees and clients in the face of an unpredictable market is my antidote to stress. I'm more alive today than I have been in the past thirty years."

When he recovered, Fisher returned to work with a new attitude toward winning. "Work has been my friend for the past two years," Fisher explained. "I threw away all my unnecessary keys (and worries)."

Fisher at one time had a huge key ring heavy with keys to the most exclusive country clubs, to boats, real estate, fancy tackle boxes, safety deposit boxes, expensive cars. He threw them all away, except the key to his present residence and a modest auto. "Keeping up with my peers and neighbors isn't worth dying for," he added.

"I paid a fortune to join the country club, but when I went there to relax after work, I drank and smoked excessively. I had a different pipe for each day of the week and enough fishing tackle for fifteen people, but I couldn't forget the office when I arrived home."

After his expensive car was stolen, Fisher dumped the keys to his clubs, boats, expensive car, and all the rest of the status symbols. "While I had my key ring, I constantly worried about how to protect and maintain the fears that keys symbolized. I panicked over how I'd acquire more money for possessions. Then I'd worry about being able to afford them. I thought my body was indestructible.

"I've changed jobs five times," Fisher added, "and each time I've had to start all over again. My stressor was the race against time, struggling longer hours against less time available to resurrect my previous income. It took a couple of heart attacks to show me that the secret of health is to make time for play and creativity on and off the job."

◆　　　◆　　　◆

Writing Health-Oriented Articles For Trade Journals Or Magazines Slanted To A Particular Type Of Industry Or Business.

Look at the health-oriented article below (on preventing hemorrhoids) that I wrote and quickly sold to a business magazine in the early 1980s (Registered Representative). The affliction has been called the plague of stock brokers. Note that the expert interviewed at the time is the author of a book on preventing hemorrhoids and at the time recounted his experience working as a stock broker.

More Than Half the People Over 42 Sitting At A Desk All Day Have Hemorrhoids

If stress-related illnesses are the leading cause of health problems, over half of sedentary middle-aged workers complain of hemorrhoids. After fifteen years of sitting in front of a desk (including a computer), Robert L. Holt left his job several years ago to write health books. He's the author of the popular book, *Hemorrhoids Cure and Prevention.* His research for the book included his experiences and the experiences of other desk-sitting workers and supervisors in his office.

"We got up around 6:00 a.m. and usually skipped breakfast to rush into the office by 7:00 a.m.," Holt explained. "We remained glued to our seats because we were afraid of missing an important message.

"Supervisors who skip breakfast and then gulp scalding coffee on an empty stomach don't have the peristalsis to move food through the intestinal tract. The normal movement of fluids is not encouraged by the lack of breakfast. Pilots have the same problem. They can't leave their seats very often, either.

"Working all day on a computer contributes to hemorrhoids as does watching ticker tape or seeing one social work client after another without taking a break. Over half the workers in my own office complained of 'rhoids. And I wasn't willing to admit then that I had them myself until I started researching hemorrhoids in medical texts."

Holt explained that, "according to a Mayo Clinic study during the sixties, out of 27,000 of their patients surveyed, 52 percent of the men and women over the age of 42 had hemorrhoids." That's the majority of people who sit most of the day at their desks. "It's probably closer to two-thirds of the population."

When I wrote this early 1980s article, I also interviewed other stock brokers working in the field. Another stock broker (named John) gave me an interview. I've left his last name out here. His comment noted what he considered to be the two major stressors in his office at that time. I wrote the following in that article:

John _____ would like to see coffee drinking and smoking decreased among office workers. He considers the two biggest stressors to be "fear of talking on the phone" and "not being well-prepared." He beats stress by talking positively to himself each morning and by being organized.

"Since I've been working inside the office," John said, "I've found I can't keep the weight off. I come in at 6:30 AM and sit at least eight hours a day." He spends at least an hour each day lifting weights.

◆   ◆   ◆

Note that when writing a medical article for a business magazine, the writer needs to emphasize what problems need to be solved in a work environment. The same would hold true for writing about a home or educational environment. What John would like to see changed in his office is an important value to include in a medical article. When writing for general consumer or inspirational magazines, focus on what needs to be changed or nourished.

4

Ghostwriting or Writing about DNA and Gene Hunters

If you're going to write healthcare or medical articles, one of the newest fields is genetics and molecular anthropology. You interview DNA specialists and gene hunters and write in plain language what the results of their research means to the average person interested in his or her own family's genetic history or ethnic and ancient history, such as where a person's DNA is found geographically today or appeared in prehistoric times.

You can interview experts for the information and read magazine articles, books, and join discussion groups on DNA and genealogy that are on the Web. Join your local university's anthropology club if it's open to the public, or join lifelong learning classes at the university campus that has an anthropology club so you can attend as a continuing education student. Some of these clubs are open to extended studies students and some anthropology and archaeology associations are national with local chapters that are community-oriented and open to the public.

Interview several gene hunters—geneticists and the genealogists who use their research to disseminate DNA-driven genealogy results and reports. Use email and phone. When you have enough quotes and comments collected for your article, consult scientific journals to find more people to interview. Do fact checking and edit your article so all the terminology is easy to understand by readers with no science background.

Define any technical term. Slant your article to the emphasis of the magazine. If you write for a genealogy magazine, fits the facts into the demographic of readers. The same article can emphasize different aspects of your interviews or research. For what type of magazine are you writing? Womens? Consumers? Historic? Science for the public? Genealogy? Business? Educational? Health? Childrens?

If you write for a magazine, ask to keep your copyright. It's worth it in the future if you want to use your material for a book. Never give up all your writes to a publisher. If you do, expect to find your article on the Web minus your byline. When you give up all your rights, your article will be copyrighted by the publisher, and no further pay will come to you. I have always kept my copyright on material that I cared for enough to want for the future.

Give an editor first time rights or one-time rights—even if it means accepting a few cents less per word. Then use your material for any other projects that may come to you in the future.

Here's a *short excerpt* from a published magazine clip of an article I wrote for one magazine, Everton's Family History PLUS, in their May/June 2004, issue on DNA-driven genealogy. The article's title is *"A Beginner's Guide to Interpreting Tests for Family History."*

Feature article

May/June 2004 Family History Magazine PLUS
www.familyhistorymagazine.com HISTORY Related Details LifeStories VitalStatistics

A Beginner's Guide to Interpreting DNA Tests for Family History

By Anne Hart

What to expect from a DNA test for ancestry

DNA testing for family history blends genealogy with biological research. "Anthrogenealogy" is Family Tree DNA's word of choice "for the study of deep genealogical origins through means of genetics." What you should expect from a DNA test for ancestry is a report on the history and geography of a few of your genes. The first step is to find out how many genetic markers will be tested before you choose a DNA testing company. Family Tree DNA offers Cohanim tests and several other ethnic and geographic origins DNA tests.

Other companies that offer similar services include Trace Genetics, <www.tracegenetics.com>; Oxford Ancestors, <www.oxfordancestors.com>; Roots for Real, <www.rootsforreal.com/english/eng-home.html>; Ancestry-ByDNA, <www.ancestrybydna.com>; Gene Tree DNA Testing Center, <www.genetree.com/about/genetree-info.asp>. There are others and you should search for the one that meets your personal needs.

Laboratories that check DNA for ancestral purposes only test markers from the D-Loop, a section of your genome that shows ancestry, not genetic risks or disease markers. Men and women have different areas of DNA tested. Because women don't have a Y-chromosome, only their maternal line—the mtDNA—can be tested.

For the maternal line, 400 base pairs of mitochondrial DNA (mtDNA) sequences are the minimum needed to perform an accurate test. Those 400 base pairs usually are all that are tested by most DNA testing companies. The 400 base pairs are required to arrive at the maternal DNA lineage haplogroup (category), which helps to point to the geographic location of your ancestry.

When testing the paternal line by Y-chromosome, 37 markers are ideal, but 25 markers also should be useful. Some companies offer a 12-marker test for surname genealogy groups at a special price that are useful only for men with the same surname from the same area, such as in a surname club looking for matching markers to indicate some relationship.

This is useful if you already have the genealogy records. For example, all of my Hart family males are listed in genealogy books back to Stephen Hart, born in 1605. In this case, a 12-marker test is helpful because we already have all the male names and the names of their wives and children.

DNA testing kits include a kit number. That number is used throughout the testing process and your name remains private. Some companies let you sign release forms to allow others to contact you by e-mail. Some companies e-mail you that you have a DNA match and you should click on the database Web site to see if others share your DNA sequences.

If you want, you can contact those who share your mtDNA and who have agreed to have their contract information released. The significance of contacting others with the same mtDNA or Y-chromosome sequence is that you know you are descended from a common relative at some point.

According to AncestryByDNA, "We've all originated from a common ancestor that lived some 200,000 years ago. The only way to know where you came from is by reading your genetic code." What might intrigue some is taking a racial percentages test to see what percentages of which "races" live in your very ancient or recent past.

What will be on the DNA Report

You'll find your sequences in letters and/or numbers on the printout that you get back from your DNA testing company, but how do you interpret your sequences for ancestry? If you want more information on interpreting sequences than you find in this article, you can start with the free online message boards on DNA genealogy such as Genealogy-DNA Rootsweb at GENEALOGY-DNA-D-request@rootsweb.com.

There are many books that can help interpret DNA test results for family history. Try The Beginner's Guide to Interpreting Ethnic DNA Origins for Family History or Creative Genealogy Projects. For more information on ancestry and DNA for genealogy buffs, try my book, Find Your Personal Adam & Eve: Make DNA-Driven Genealogy Time Capsules.

The book also explains how nutritional genetics testing and DNA testing for ancestry interacts, and how food and medicines reveal your genetic signature or expression. Call toll free, 877.823.9235 or visit <www.iuniverse.com>. Available for download on my Web site are instructional videos on interpreting your DNA test results for family history and ancestry. Do your research before you take a DNA test, because your biggest question could be how to apply DNA sequence interpretations to the field of genealogy.

What you will pay for a DNA test for ancestry

In August 2001, Oxford Ancestors, located in London, became the first company to test my mtDNA for around $180. They noted that my mtDNA sequences showed up in England. They sent me a chart showing where the mtDNA originated and how my mtDNA links with other mtDNA all over the world. I received printed material on human migrations. I paid a little more than $200 at Family Tree DNA. I had my mtDNA tested again to find out the high-resolution mtDNA (called the HVR-2). With both the high and low mtDNA results, there's a better chance of finding closer DNA matches who are possible relatives. My husband paid $99 for a surname group-rate 12-marker Y-chromosome test at Family Tree DNA.

At most companies, DNA tests for ancestry cost from about $100 to more than $300. Prices seem to be coming down and more markers are being tested for Y-chromosomes. DNA tests for nutrition or medical reasons are more expensive, and a few companies even test the entire genome, though the price is usually more than $1,000.

How to interpret DNA test results—Female

Ancestors, a DNA testing group, refers to the haplogroup as a "clan" (because it's easier to remember). If you're of European, Middle Eastern, or from some parts of India, your deep maternal ancestry letters will be H, I, J, K, N, R, T, U, V, W or X. Most European lineages of women have these letters. It only means your prehistoric female ancestors most likely came from Europe, Central Asia or the Middle East.

If your letters are A, B, C, D or X, it is most likely you could be Native American or Asian. The letter "L" is African, and the letters M, A, B, C, D, E, F, G, O, P, Q and Z most likely are East Asian. A and C are shared by East Asian and Native American, and Z is occasionally found in Russia and Scandinavia. These haplogroups are ancient. Some extend back 20,000 years or more than 50,000 years into prehistory.

If your mtDNA indicates a wide area, it usually signifies that the DNA sequences are very ancient and had thousands of years to spread large distances geographically. If your mtDNA sequences are found in a very limited area, your mtDNA may have arisen relatively recently. Your DNA's geographic place of origin is the land where your DNA sequences are most diverse, not necessarily where it is found most frequently. For example, my mtDNA is most diverse in northern India, central Asia and Iraq. Those are likely places where my maternal DNA originated, even though it has dwelled in northern Europe for several thousand years and is found most frequently in Europe today.

Where you can match your mtDNA to a country in an online database

For women and men interested in matching their mtDNA sequences of HVS-1 or HVS-2 (high and low resolution) there are databases online such as Macaulay's Tables database. These online DNA databases are matched with surname groups, lists, message boards and other Web databases to help match your sequences to a geographic location. I use Macaulay's Tables at <www.stats.gla.ac.uk/~vincent/founder2000/tableA.html>.

Roots for Real is based in London. This company tests your low-resolution mtDNA or Y-chromosome and sends you a report and map showing the probable or possible geographic origin of your sequence by latitude and longitude, even naming the town that exists there today. The probable geographic center for the origin of my mtDNA sequences is located at 48.30N, 4.65E, Bar sur Aube, France, with a deviation of 669.62 miles according to the map e-mailed to me by Roots for Real.

How to interpret DNA test results—Males

Males take Y-chromosome DNA tests to find out paternal ancestry lineages. Males also can have their mtDNA checked. Women don't have a Y-chromosome, so women can only check their maternal lineages with mitochondrial (mtDNA) tests. Women who want to check their paternal lineage need only find a direct male relative—one who is descended from the woman's father, paternal grandfather, paternal great-grandfather or father's brothers—who is willing to provide a DNA sample.

Looking for more?

Family Tree DNA—Genealogy by Genetics Ltd.
World Headquarters, 1919 North Loop W., Suite 110, Houston, TX 77008
http://www.familytreedna.com

AncestryByDNA
DNAPrint Genomics Inc., 900 Cocoanut Ave., Sarasota, FL 34236 http://www.ancestrybydna.com/

Oxford Ancestors
Oxford Ancestors Ltd., P.O. Box 288, Kidlington OX5 1WB United Kingdom
http://www.oxfordancestors.com

Roots for Real
P.O. Box 43708, London W14 8WG United Kingdom
http://www.rootsforreal.com/english/contact.html
E-mail: info@rootsforreal.com

GeneTree DNA Testing Center
2495 South West Temple
Salt Lake City, UT 84115 http://www.genetree.com/

Trace Genetics LLC
P.O. Box 2010
Davis, California 95617
http://www.tracegenetics.com/aboutus.html info@tracegenetics.com

Predictive Genomics for Personalized Medicine including Nutrigenomics
AlphaGenics Inc.
9700 Great Seneca Highway
Rockville,   Maryland   20850   http://www.alpha-genics.com/index.php
info@alpha-genics.com

Genovations ™ Great Smokies Diagnostic Laboratory/Genovations™
63 Zillicoa Street
Asheville, NC 28801 USA http://www.genovations.com/

Centre for Human Nutrigenomics http://www.nutrigenomics.nl/
According to its Web site, "The Centre for Human NutriGenomics aims at establishing an international centre of expertise combining excellent pre-competitive research and high quality (post)graduate training on the interface of genomics, nutrition and human health."

Nutrigenomics Links: http://nutrigene.4t.com/nutrigen.htm
Veterinary Genetics Laboratory
University of California, Davis
One Shields Avenue
Davis, CA 95616-8744 http://www.vgl.ucdavis.edu/

DNA Testing of Dogs and Horses
VetGen, 3728 Plaza Drive, Suite 1, Ann Arbor, Michigan, 48108 USA http://www.vetgen.com/

◆   ◆   ◆

Medical writers can also prepare articles on for entrepreneurial magazines on the business end of running a DNA reporting service. Here's a sample article on how to start and operate a business compiling DNA test results in plain language. A reporting service would act as a liaison between the DNA testing laboratory and the genealogy firm or genealogist working directly with clients.

Your job as a medical writer and independent contractor would be to explain in print and/or on CDs or DVDs what the results mean to someone without any science background. You might call this applied predictive medicine journalism or publishing. Another alternative would be to work in multimedia, putting results on DVDs or CDs as well as offering a text copy.

You'd be a writer and a publisher, preparing reports for companies that do DNA testing. The reports would be in plain language with all terms and results clearly explained. You'd find the answers by interviewing experts and finding out what the results mean and how the client applies them. You'd work with genetic counselors, physicians trained in interpreting DNA tests for risks or for ancestry.

Your job as a writer or publisher would be to put into plain language the results that go to the client, the person who has had his or her DNA tested—either for ancestry and genealogy or for disease predisposition and genetic risk.

Either way, your writing is confidential and private. You'd communicate with the testing laboratory, the interpreting physician and/or genetics counselor, any other experts consulted, and the client—always keeping the results private and confidential, whether for ancestry purposes or (a completely different DNA test) for predisposition and risk.

Are You Interested in DNA Results Reporting or Book Packaging and Information Disseminating? Here's How to Open Your Own DNA Test Results or Molecular Genealogy Reporting Company

Did you ever wonder what the next money-making step for entrepreneurs in genealogy is—searching records for family history and ancestry? It's about opening a genealogy-driven DNA testing service. Take your pick: tracking ancestry by DNA for pets or people. You don't need any science courses or degrees to start or operate this small business. It can be done online, at home, or in an office.

What should you charge per test? About $200 is affordable. You'll have to pay a laboratory to do the testing. Work out your budget with the laboratory.

Laboratories that do the testing can take up to fifty percent of what you make on each test unless they have research grants to test a particular ethnic group and need donors to give DNA for testing. Each lab is different. Shop around for an affordable, reputable laboratory.

Your first step would be to ask the genetics and/or molecular anthropology departments of universities who's applying for a grant to do DNA testing. Also check out the oral history libraries which usually are based at universities and ethnic museums. You're bringing together two different groups—genealogists and geneticists.

You'd work with the laboratories that do the testing. Customers want to see online message boards to discuss their DNA test results and find people whose DNA sequences match their own.

So you'd need a Web site with databases of the customers, message boards, and any type of interactive communication system that allows privacy and communication. DNA database material would not show real names or identify the people. So you'd use numbers. Those who want to contact others could use regular email addresses. People want ethnic privacy, but at the same time love to find DNA matches. At this point you might want to work only with dogs, horses, or other pets or farm animals providing a DNA testing service for ancestry or nutrition.

Take your choice as an entrepreneur: sending the DNA of people to laboratories to be tested for ancestry or having the DNA of dogs, horses or other pets and animals sent out to be tested for ancestry and supplying reports to owners regarding ancestry or for information on how to tailor food to the genetic signatures of people or animals. For animals, you'd contact breeders.

For people, your next step is to contact genealogists and genealogy online and print publications. You'd focus on specific ethnic groups as a niche market. The major groups interested in ancestry using DNA testing include Northern European, Ashkenazi, Italian, Greek, Armenian, Eastern European, African, Asian, Latin American, and Middle Eastern.

Many successful entrepreneurs in the DNA testing for ancestry businesses started with a hobby of looking up family history records—genealogy. So if you're a history buff, or if your hobby is family history research, oral history, archaeology, or genealogy, you now can turn to DNA testing.

What you actually sell to customers are DNA test kits and DNA test reports. To promote your business, offer free access to your Web site database with all your clients listed by important DNA sequences. Keep names private and use only assigned numbers or letters to protect the privacy of your clients. Never give private and confidential genetic test information to insurance companies or employers. Clients who want to have their DNA tested for ancestry do not want their names and DNA stored to fall into the "wrong hands." So honor privacy requests. Some people will actually ask you to store DNA for future generations.

If you want to include this service, offer a time capsule. For your clients, you would create a time capsule, which is like a secure scrap book on acid-free paper and on technology that can be transferred in the future when technology changes. Don't store anything on materials that can't be transferred from one technology to another. For example, have reports on acid-free paper.

You can include a CD or DVD also, but make sure that in the future when the CD players aren't around any longer, the well-preserved report, perhaps laminated or on vellum or other acid-free materials that don't crumble with age can be put into the time capsule. You can include a scrap book with family photos and video on a CD if you wish, or simply offer the DNA test report and comments explaining to the customer what the DNA shows.

Use plain language and no technical terms unless you define them on the same page. Your goal is to help people find other people who match DNA sequences and to use this knowledge to send your customers reports. If no matches can be found, then supply your clients with a thorough report. Keep out any confusing jargon. Show with illustrations how your customer's DNA was tested. In plain language tell them what was done.

Your report will show the results, and tell simply what the results mean. You can offer clients a list of how many people in what countries have their same DNA sequences. Include the present day city or town and the geographic location using longitude and latitude. For example, when I had my mtDNA (maternal lineages) tested, the report included my DNA matches by geographic coordinates. The geographic center is 48.30N 4.65E, Bar sur Aube, France with a deviation of 669.62 miles as done by "Roots for Real," a London company that tests DNA for ancestry. The exact sequences are in the Roots for Real Database (and other mtDNA databases) for my markers.

You're going to ask, with no science background yourself, how will you know what to put in the report? That's the second step. You contact a university laboratory that does DNA testing for outside companies. They will generate all the reports for you. What you do with the report is to promote it by making it look visually appealing. Define any words you think the customer won't understand with simpler words that fully explain what the DNA sequences mean and what the various letters and numbers mean. Any dictionary of genetic terms will give you the meaning in one sentence using plain language. Use short sentences in your reports and plain language.

Your new service targets genealogists who help their own customers find lost relatives. Your secondary market is the general public. Most people taking a DNA test for ancestry want information on where their DNA roamed 20,000 years ago and in the last 10,000 years. DNA testing shows people only where their ancient ancestors camped. However, when sequences with other people match exactly, it could point the way to an ancient common ancestor whose descendants went in a straight line from someone with those sequences who lived 10,000 years ago to a common ancestor who lived only a few generations ago.

Those people may or may not actually be related, but they share the same sequences. The relationship could be back in a straight line 20,000 years or more or only a few centuries. Ancient DNA sequences are spread over a huge area, like mine—from Iceland to Bashkortostan in the Urals. DNA sequences that sprung up only a few generations ago generally are limited to a more narrow geographic area, except for those who lived in isolation in one area for thousands of years, such as the Basques.

You would purchase wholesale DNA kits from laboratory suppliers and send the kits to your customer. The customer takes a painless cheek scraping with a felt or cotton type swab or uses mouthwash put into a small container to obtain DNA that can help accurately determine a relationship with either a 99.9% probability of YES or a 100% certainly that no near term relationship existed.

The DNA sample is sealed and mailed to a laboratory address where it is tested. The laboratory then disposes of the DNA after a report is generated. Then you package the report like a gift card portfolio, a time capsule, or other fancy packaging to look like a gift. You add your promotional material and a thorough explanation of what to expect from the DNA test—the results.

The best way to learn this business is to check out on the Web all the businesses that are doing this successfully. Have your own DNA tested and look at the printout or report of the results. Is it thorough? Does it eliminate jargon? Include in the report materials the client would like to see. Make it look like a press kit. For example, you take a folder such as a report folder. On the outside cover print the name of your company printed and a logo or photograph of something related to DNA that won't frighten away the consumer. Simple graphic art such as a map or globe of the world, a prehistoric statue, for example the Willendorf Venus, or some other symbol is appropriate.

Inside, you'd have maps, charts, and locations for the client to look at. Keep the material visual. Include a CD with the DNA sequences if you can. The explanation would show the customer the steps taken to test the DNA.

Keep that visual with charts and graphs. Don't use small print fonts or scientific terminology to any extent so your customer won't feel your report is over his or her head. Instead use illustrations, geographic maps. Put colorful circles on the cities or geographic locations where that person's DNA is found.

Put a bright color or arrow on the possible geographic area of origin for those DNA sequences. Nobody can pinpoint an exact town for certain, but scientists know where certain DNA sequences are found and where they might have sat out the last Ice Age 20,000 years ago, and survived to pass those same DNA sequences on to their direct descendants, that customer of yours who has those sequences.

In the last decade, businesses have opened offering personality profilers. This decade, since the human genome code was cracked and scientists know a lot more about DNA testing for the courtroom, DNA testing businesses have opened to test DNA for information other than who committed a crime or to prove who's innocent. Applications of DNA testing now are used for finding ancient and not-so-ancient ancestry. DNA testing is not only used for paternity and maternity testing, but for tailoring what you eat to your genetic signature. The new field of pharmacogenetics also tests DNA for markers that allow a client to customize medicine to his or her genetic expression.

You may be an entrepreneur with no science background. That's okay as long as your laboratory contacts are scientists. Your most important contact and contract would be with a DNA testing laboratory. Find out who your competitors contract with as far as testing laboratories. For example, Family Tree DNA at the Web site: http://www.familytreedna.com/faq.html#q1 sends its DNA samples to be tested by the DNA testing laboratories at the University of Arizona.

Bennett Greenspan, President and CEO of Family Tree DNA founded Family Tree in 1999. Greenspan is an entrepreneur and life-long genealogy enthusiast. He successfully turned his family history and ancestry hobby into a full-time vocation running a DNA testing-for-ancestry company. Together with Max Blankfeld, they founded in 1997 GoCollege.com a website for college-bound students which survived the .COM implosion. Max Blankfeld is Greenspan's Vice President of Operations/Marketing. Before entering the business world, Blankfeld was a journalist. After that, he started and managed several successful ventures in the area of public relations as well as consumer goods both in Brazil and the US. Today, the highly successful Family Tree DNA is America's first genealogy-driven DNA testing service.

At the University of Arizona, top DNA research scientists such as geneticist, Mike Hammer, PhD, population geneticist Bruce Walsh, PhD, geneticist Max F. Rothschild, molecular anthropologist, Theodore G. Schurr, and lab manager, Matthew Kaplan along with the rest of the DNA testing team do the testing and analysis.

So it's important if you want to open your own DNA for ancestry testing company to contract with a reputable laboratory to do the testing. Find out whether the lab you're going to be dealing with will answer a client's questions in case of problems with a test that might require re-testing. Clients will come to you to answer questions rather than go to the busy laboratory. Most laboratories are either part of a university, a medical school, or are independent DNA testing laboratories run by scientists and their technicians and technologists.

Your business will have a very different focus if you're only dealing with genealogy buffs testing their DNA for ancestry than would a business testing DNA for genetic risk markers in order to tailor a special diet or foods to someone's genetic risk markers. For that more specialized business, you'd have to partner with a nutritionist, scientist, or physician trained in customizing diets to genetic signatures. Many independent laboratories do test genes for the purpose of tailoring diets to genes. The new field is called nutrigenomics. Check out the various Web sites devoted to nutrigenomics if you're interested in this type of DNA testing business. For example, there is Alpha-Genetics at http:// www.Alpha-Genics.com.

According to Dr. Fredric D. Abramson, PhD, S.M., President and CEO of AlphaGenics, Inc., "The key to using diet to manage genes and health lies in managing gene expression (which we call the Expressitype). Knowing your geno-type merely tells you a starting point. Genotype is like knowing where the entrance ramps to an interstate can be found.

They are important to know, but tell you absolutely nothing about what direction to travel or how the journey will go. That is why Expressitype must be the focus." You can contact AlphaGenics, Inc. at: http:// www.Alpha-Genics.com or write to: Maryland Technology Incubator, 9700 Great Seneca Highway, Rockville, MD 20850.

Why open any kind of a DNA testing business? It's because the entrepreneur is at the forefront of a revolution in our concept of ancestry, diet, and medicines. Genes are tested to reveal how your body metabolizes medicine as well as food, and genes are tested for ancient ancestry or recent relationships such as paternity. Genes are tested for courtroom evidence.

You have the choice of opening a DNA testing service focusing on diet, ancestry, skin care product matches, or medicine. You can have scientists contract with you to test genes for risk or relationships. Some companies claim to test DNA in order to determine whether the skin care products are right for your genetic signature. It goes beyond the old allergy tests of the eighties.

"Each of us is a unique organism, and for the first time in human history, genetic research is confirming that one diet is not optimum for everyone," says Abramson. Because your genes differ from someone else's, you process food and supplements in a unique way. Your ancestry is unique also.

Do you want to open a business that tunes nutrition to meet the optimum health needs of each person? If so, you need to contract with scientists to do the testing. If you have no science background, it would be an easier first step to open a business that tests DNA only for ancestry and contract with university laboratories who know about genes and ancestry.

Your client would receive a report on only the ancestry. This means the maternal and/or paternal sequences. For a woman it's the mtDNA that's tested. You're testing the maternal lineages. It's ancient and goes back thousands of years. For the man, you can have a lab test the Y-chromosome, the paternal lineages and the mtDNA, the maternal lineages.

What you supply your clients with is a printout report and explanation of the individual's sequences and mtDNA group called the haplogroup and/or the Y-chromosome ancestral genetic markers. For a male, you can test the Y-chromosome and provide those markers, usually 25 markers and the mtDNA. For a woman, you can only test the mtDNA, the maternal line for haplogroup letter and what is called the HVS-1 and HVS-2 sequences. These sequences show the maternal lineages back thousands of years. To get started, look at the Web sites and databases of all the companies that test for ancestry using DNA.

What most of the DNA testing entrepreneurs have in common is that they can do business online. People order the DNA testing kit online. The companies send out a DNA testing kit. The client sends back DNA to a lab to be tested. The process does not involve any blood drawing to test for ancestry. Then the company sends a report directly to the customer about what the DNA test revealed solely in regard to ancient ancestry—maternal or paternal lines.

Reports include the possible geographic location where the DNA sequences originated. Customers usually want to see the name of an actual town, even though towns didn't exist 10,000 years ago when the sequences might have arisen. The whole genome is not tested, only the few ancestral markers, usually 500 base pairs of genes. Testing DNA for ancestry does not have anything to do with testing genes for health risks because only certain genes are tested—genes related to ancestry. And all the testing is done at a laboratory, not at your online business.

If you're interested in a career in genetics counseling and wish to pursue a graduate degree in genetics counseling, that's another career route. For information, contact The American Board of Genetic Counseling. Sometimes social workers with some coursework in biology take a graduate degree in genetic counseling since it combines counseling skills with training in genetics and in interpreting genetics tests for your clients.

The American Board of Genetic Counseling
9650 Rockville Pike
Bethesda, MD 20814-3998
http://www.abgc.net/

Predictive Genomics for Personalized Medicine including Nutrigenomics
AlphaGenics Inc.

9700 Great Seneca Highway
Rockville, Maryland 20850
Email: info@alpha-genics.com
http://www.alpha-genics.com/index.php

Genovations ™
Great Smokies Diagnostic Laboratory/Genovations™
63 Zillicoa Street
Asheville, NC 28801 USA
http://www.genovations.com/

Centre for Human Nutrigenomics
http://www.nutrigenomics.nl/
According to its Web site, "The Centre for Human NutriGenomics aims at establishing an international centre of expertise combining excellent pre-competitive research and high quality (post)graduate training on the interface of genomics, nutrition and human health."

Nutrigenomics Links: http://nutrigene.4t.com/nutrigen.htm

Veterinary DNA Testing

Veterinary Genetics Laboratory
University of California, Davis
One Shields Avenue
Davis, CA 95616-8744
http://www.vgl.ucdavis.edu/

According to their Web site: "The Veterinary Genetics Laboratory is internationally recognized for its expertise in parentage verification and genetic diagnostics for animals. VGL has provided services to breed registries, practitioners, individual owners and breeders since 1955." The Veterinary Genetics Laboratory performs contracted DNA testing.
Alpaca/Llama
Beefalo
Cat
Cattle
Dog

Elk
Goat
Horse
Sheep

DNA Testing of Dogs and Horses
VetGen, 3728 Plaza Drive, Suite 1, Ann Arbor, Michigan, 48108 USA http://
www.vetgen.com/

◆   ◆   ◆

Ethnic Genealogy Web Sites

(Usually, there are several genealogy sites on the Web for each ethnic group.)

Acadian/Cajun: & French Canadian: http://www.acadian.org/tidbits.html
Afghanistan Genealogy: http://www.kindredtrails.com/afghanistan.html
African-American: http://www.cyndislist.com/african.htm
African Royalty Genealogy: http://www.uq.net.au/~zzhsoszy/
Albanian Research List: http://feefhs.org/al/alrl.html
Armenian Genealogical Society: http://feefhs.org/am/frg-amgs.html
Asia and the Pacific: http://www.cyndislist.com/asia.htm
Austria-Hungary Empire: http://feefhs.org/ah/indexah.html
Baltic-Russian Information Center: http://feefhs.org/blitz/frgblitz.html
Belarusian—Association of the Belarusian Nobility: http://feefhs.org/by/frg-zbs.html
Bukovina Genealogy: http://feefhs.org/bukovina/bukovina.html
Carpatho-Rusyn Knowledge Base: http://feefhs.org/rusyn/frg-crkb.html
Chinese Genealogy: http://www.chineseroots.com.
Croatia Genealogy Cross Index: http://feefhs.org/cro/indexcro.html
Czechoslovak Genealogical Society Int'l, Inc.: http://feefhs.org/czs/cgsi/frg-cgsi.html
Eastern Europe: http://www.cyndislist.com/easteuro.htm
Eastern European Genealogical Society, Inc.: http://feefhs.org/ca/frg-eegs.html
Eastern Europe Ethnic, Religious, and National Index with Home Pages includes the FEEFHS Resource Guide that lists organizations associated

with FEEFHS from 14 Countries. It also includes Finnish and Armenian genealogy resources: http://feefhs.org/ ethnic.html

Ethnic, Religious, and National Index 14 countries: http://feefhs.org/ethnic.html

(Finland) Genealogical Society of Finland: http://www.genealogia.fi/indexe.htm

Finnish Genealogy Group: http://feefhs.org/misc/frgfinmn.html

Galicia Jewish SIG: http://feefhs.org/jsig/frg-gsig.html

German Genealogical Digest: http://feefhs.org/pub/frg-ggdp.html

Greek Genealogy Sources on the Internet: http://www-personal.umich.edu/~cgaunt/greece.html

Genealogy Societies Online List: http://www.daddezio.com/catalog/grkndx04.html

German Research Association: http://feefhs.org/gra/frg-gra.html

Greek Genealogy (Hellenes-Diaspora Greek Genealogy): http://www.geocities. com/SouthBeach/Cove/4537/

Greek Genealogy Home Page: http://www.daddezio.com/grekgen.html

Greek Genealogy Articles: http://www.daddezio.com/catalog/grkndx01.html

India Genealogy: http://genforum.genealogy.com/india/

India Family Histories: http://www.mycinnamontoast.com/perl/results.cgi?region=79&sort=n

India-Anglo-Indian/Europeans in India genealogy: http://members.ozemail.com.au/~clday/

Irish Travelers: http://www.pitt.edu/~alkst3/Traveller.html

Japanese Genealogy: http://www.rootsweb.com/~jpnwgw/

Jewish Genealogy: http://www.jewishgen.org/infofiles/

Latvian Jewish Genealogy Page: http://feefhs.org/jsig/frg-lsig.html

Lebanese Genealogy: http://www.rootsweb.com/~lbnwgw/

Lithuanian American Genealogy Society: http://feefhs.org/frg-lags.html

Melungeon: http://www.geocities.com/Paris/5121/melungeon.htm

Mennonite Heritage Center: http://feefhs.org/men/frg-mhc.html

Middle East Genealogy: http://www.rootsweb.com/~mdeastgw/index.html

Middle East Genealogy by country: http://www.rootsweb.com/~mdeastgw/index.html#country

Native American: http://www.cyndislist.com/native.htm

Polish Genealogical Society of America: http://feefhs.org/pol/frg-pgsa.html

Quebec and Francophone: http://www.francogene.com/quebec/amerin.html

Romanian American Heritage Center: http://feefhs.org/ro/frg-rahc.html

Slovak World: http://feefhs.org/slovak/frg-sw.html

Slavs, South: Cultural Society: http://feefhs.org/frg-csss.html

Syrian and Lebanese Genealogy: http://www.genealogytoday.com/family/syrian/

Syria Genealogy: http://www.rootsweb.com/~syrwgw/

Tibetan Genealogy: http://www.distantcousin.com/Links/Ethnic/China/Tibetan.html

Turkish Genealogy Discussion Group: http://www.turkey.com/forums/forumdisplay.php3?forumid=18

Ukrainian Genealogical and Historical Society of Canada: http://feefhs.org/ca/frgughsc.html

Unique Peoples: http://www.cyndislist.com/peoples.htm **Note: The Unique People's list includes: Black Dutch, Doukhobors, Gypsy, Romani, Romany & Travellers, Melungeons, Metis, Miscellaneous, and Wends/Sorbs Genealogy, (General):**

Ancestry.com: http://www.ancestry.com/main.htm?lfl=m

BMD Certificates, London, England, UK: http://www.bmd-certificates.co.uk

Cyndi's List of Genealogy on the Internet: http://www.cyndislist.com/

Cyndi's List is a categorized & cross-referenced index to genealogical resources on the Internet with thousands of links.

DistantCousin.com (Uniting Cousins Worldwide) http://distantcousin.com/Links/surname.html

Ellis Island Online: http://www.ellisisland.org/

Family History Library: http://www.familysearch.org/Eng/default.asp http://www.familysearch.org/Eng/Search/frameset_search.asp

(The Church of Jesus Christ of Latter Day Saints) International Genealogical Index

Female Ancestors: http://www.cyndislist.com/female.htm

Genealogist's Index to the Web: http://www.genealogytoday.com/GIWWW/?

Genealogy Web: http://www.genealogyweb.com/

Genealogy Authors and Speakers: http://feefhs.org/frg/frg-a&l.html

Genealogy Today: http://www.genealogytoday.com/

My Genealogy.com: http://www.genealogy.com/cgi-bin/my_main.cgi

Scriver, Dr. Charles: The Canadian Medical Hall of Fame http://www.virtualmuseum.ca/Exhibitions/Medicentre/en/scri_print.htm

Surname Sites: http://www.cyndislist.com/surn-gen.htm

National Genealogical Society: http://www.ngsgenealogy.org/index.htm

United States List of Local by State Genealogical Societies: http://www.dad dezio.com/society/hill/index.html
United States Vital Records List: http://www.daddezio.com/records/room/ index.html **or** http://www.cyndislist.com/usvital.htm

5

Ghostwriting the Self-Help Article

Do your press/media releases for published self-help articles answer the question **what, who, where, when, how, and why?** Five of those are straight news for press releases. The "why" is good for a feature article, but may be included in straight news releases. These questions are answered in order of their importance, with the most important information up front. That's called the inverted pyramid method of news writing.

The Seven C's of Communication are:
1. Credibility
2. Context
3. Content
4. Clarity
5. Continuity and Consistency
6. Channels
7. Capability of the Audience

Content and credibility as the two most important.

Content: Did you convey your message?
Credibility/Visibility/Trust

Medical writers can also find a career selling the products about which they write. Writers also can do public speaking on their research, travel, and published writing. At the same time medical journalists also can sell (or represent) the product discussed in the research and writing. It's a personal choice and often involves travel for research and reporting. It's all about sharing meaning—communication with prospective buyers of a product for some medical journalists who do enjoy public speaking.

Here is a sample of a self-help article. Note that it emphasizes the solution to a problem and results obtained by specific step-by-step answers that readers can customize and follow depending upon their own situations and individual bodies and needs.

The focus in this article is how to safely stretch muscles to relieve anxiety and what type of changes in nutrition helped one individual. Readers should always be told their needs would be different and that they should check with their physicians before attempting any type of exercise or nutrition program.

In this type of article, you're only stating what worked best for you and not advising others to do the same. Your experience is meant as an example to inspire and motivate the reader to seek individual solutions by working with his or her healthcare team. What you're offering in this type of article are alternatives and possibilities to consider exploring in conjunction with regular healthcare practices.

You're introducing the reader to research alternative solutions to problems by illustrating step-by-step what worked only for you. Explain why it worked, how it worked, and what resulted. Articles need to include answers to the questions who, what, where, why, how and when, always emphasizing that this worked for you but may not be the answer for another person.

Your objective in writing the personal experience self-help article for the healthcare field is that you're stating how you explored the alternatives and possibilities, how those alternatives worked for you and why they worked. Note that this solution to a problem reflects your individual genetic response, signature, and expression. Remember that you're not giving medical or legal advice.

Instead, you're reporting your personal experience and offering educational material and further resources for the reader to research. This type of self-help article in medical writing is called the personal experience article or significant life story event that includes how you solved your own problem and achieved results. Similar articles could be about weight loss or gain, navigating crises, or dealing with situations that some, many, or all experience moving through the various stages and ages.

Do your query letters and media releases answer the question 'what'? You'll have to sell your writing. Technical writers also sometimes work as sales representatives for the products made by the corporations whose marketing communications personnel and technical experts they interview.

Stretch Your Panic Away
How Yoga, Lifestyle, and Nutrition Changes 'Cured' My Agoraphobia with Panic Disorder

Between 1965 and early 1972 I was housebound with agoraphobia and panic disorder after the birth of my first and second children in March 1965 and in November 1966. More than two million people in the United States suffer from this incapacitating anxiety, a panic state, when traveling away from their homes. It's a fear that wells up when under even the slightest stress or in an unfamiliar situation.

When traditional medicine failed to help, a friend sent me a book on Yoga exercises and meditation. I practiced the positions with determination to help myself.

In addition to the approximately 28 Yoga postures, I used music therapy—calming ethnic music of strings, flutes, and slow drums at 60 beats per minute to bring down my naturally high adrenaline state. I also changed my diet to vegetarian, cutting out all white sugar and salted foods, all caffeine and chocolate.

My monthly "estrogen migraines" also grew less painful as a result. The vitamins I took were Vitamin E with 100 mg. of Selenium, Vitamin C, and beta carotene, and the usual B complex vitamins found in health food stores in "normal" amounts (75-100 mg.). I also took magnesium 300 and calcium 600-1000.

At the time I was 25 years old. I'm 63 now. I couldn't exercise much with agoraphobia because exercise increased the lactic acid in my body. Lactic acid creates panic attacks in persons prone to panic disorder. Exercising caused exercise asthma, hyperventilation syndrome, and panic attacks.

During pregnancy, the estrogen and progesterone levels increase dramatically in a woman's body. A pregnant woman has 200 times as much estrogen in her body than before or after pregnancy.

After childbirth, that estrogen level drops suddenly. For me, the result was panic attacks with agoraphobia and hyperventilation syndrome.

The only way to get rid of my fear of leaving the house and the panic attacks was to get pregnant again. By the third month of pregnancy I'd feel incredibly calm again. But I couldn't do that forever, especially when my first husband divorced me after the second child.

Yoga required stretching instead of the usual exercise movement that would increase my already hyper state of adrenaline and insulin in my blood. In addition, I had low blood sugar (hypoglycemia). My fasting blood glucose of 86 would drop to 60 when I drank two tablespoons of honey in lemon water during a glucose tolerance test.

In short, for seven years I was totally housebound and suffered dozens of panic attacks a day some days. Other days I'd only have chronic anxiety for the entire day....and panic when I had to sit in a classroom. At the time I was an evening school graduate student. I'd tried every exercise from aerobics to belly dancing.

Yoga was the only movement that relaxed me. The stretching of my muscles removed the lactic acid from my body in the same way that a runner stretches a leg against a tree to cool down and remove the lactic acid that builds up in the body during exercise.

Persons who are biologically prone to agoraphobia and panic under the slightest stress normally are born with shy, over-aroused (dominant introverted feeling) nervous systems. They secrete a high level of catecholamine. Their adrenaline level is always at a higher base level than in the average or naturally calm person. They secrete more insulin into their blood that people who are literally immune from anxiety attacks.

I'd been a person with an avoidant/dependent personality type. I withdrew from direct people contact and became a recluse in order to stop being a "hot reactor." A hot reactor reacts to the slightest stress by a dramatically increased blood pressure, pulse rate, and sudden, gripping fear to people and slight mental stress.

As a biological introvert, sensitive to people's actions, noise, intrusions, and words, my whole body would over react to any stress in my environment, until I had to back off and become housebound.

I couldn't work at any job that brought me into contact with people directly. The phone would ring and my pulse and pressure would hit the ceiling. I didn't dare answer the phone or I'd go into hyperventilation syndrome and start breathing too fast in terror at the voice on the other end. I was expending a ton of energy in response to an ounce of provocation. I was afraid of everything that could elicit a physiological response in me.

To counteract my weak calming branch, the more I stretched with Yoga exercises, the cooler and calmer I became. I noticed that at the height of my panic attack, I'd go into the Yoga positions and stretch my muscles. The result was a sudden sense of calm.

The anxiety would fade. A feeling of sending out waves of love to my worst enemy took over my body and mind. My dominant introverted feeling personality type emphasized values. I asked myself: Is this issue worth weakening my heart's pacemaker by an adrenaline bath? The answer was always, of course not. Now, my body had to understand that feeling value at the molecular level as well.

Also of help were the calming, meditative new age and ethnic music that relaxed me. My whole body would physiologically react to the beat of the music. The slow beats brought me down. Music distracted my brain from firing off anxiety neurons.

The right hemisphere of my brain was shooting off energy from neurons a lot faster that the left hemisphere of my brain when the both hemispheres should have been working together in balance at more or less the same rate. This was another cause of my chronic anxiety, panic attacks, and ultimately being housebound with agoraphobia (literally, fear of the outdoors).

What I was really afraid of was not "the marketplace, or outdoors (agora in Greek), but my body's panic reaction to stress.

I perceived stress as threatening so fast that my logical side didn't have time to calm myself down. I had a weak calming branch.

Again Yoga came to the rescue. How Yoga worked specifically was by the actual stretching of the muscles. When muscles stretch they cool down the panic by changing the posture. The stretching removed the adrenaline, lactic acid, and insulin from the muscles, and the muscles stopped shaking.

My breathing grew slower as I stretched and went through the basic postures. My migraines eased. Meditation became easier. Finally, I could relax afterward.

To get rid of the panic attack, I'd begin by sitting in a half-lotus position. For hyperventilation syndrome, I'd breathe into a brown paper bag to increase the carbon dioxide. However, when I was back to normal, I'd breathe fresh air slowly because carbon dioxide causes sensitive people with panic disorder to have a panic attack from breathing carbon dioxide.

Then I'd hold my left foot firmly and place my left foot and heel against my right mid-thigh while stretching my arms downward. Then I'd reverse and place my right foot against the inside of my left thigh and gently stretch. An almost immediate feeling of calming ensued.

The position with my right foot resting and stretching against my left thigh is what calmed me more than the position of my left foot against my right thigh. I stretched as many muscles as I could easily stretch and then relaxed. I let my forearm relax and rest against my raised knee. I'd sit for two minutes in this posture.

The weight of my forearm gradually lowered my knee. By the time the knee was lowered as far as it needed to go, I calmed down. Slow deep breathing was very helpful.

Yoga also helped my inner ear problems. I have a damaged left inner ear that caused vertigo attacks whenever I was under stress.

The stretching and movement of yoga basic postures helped me regain my balance. Eventually my brain compensated for the damaged inner ear, and the vertigo and ear problems lessened, especially by the side bend Yoga exercise.

I'd recommend any person housebound by agoraphobia to start a Yoga regimen backed up by balanced nutrition, vitamins and minerals, and meditation with music therapy. Of all the therapies I tried, Yoga worked the best. Years later, I practice Yoga combined with slow belly dancing and Tai Chi Chuan, meditation, slow beat ethnic, new age, and classical music, and of course, the right foods of whole grains and legumes, fresh and juiced vegetables, and no sugar or excessive salt.

My motto is stretching your panic away. I'd take this regimen anytime over addictive tranquilizers, addictive drugs with side effects, or antidepressants that do nothing for the panic, but treat the depression that are usually prescribed for agoraphobia with panic disorder. I didn't feel depressed. I felt scared out of my skin, scared to tremors. The seizure of shaking felt almost like a mild epileptic set of convulsions. Yet, I was always told after seeing dozens of doctors that nothing showed up on tests.

Back then in 1965, my doctors told me my panic attacks were all in my head, and I was in good health. They automatically gave me a prescription for Miltown or Librium. When I got older and complained of too much adrenaline in my blood, they gave me a prescription for Inderal, a beta blocker to stop adrenalin from hitting my heart's electrical system.

Over the years, I'd developed arrhythmias which I helped with the correct dosage of fish oils containing Omega 3 fatty acids, 150 mg. of selenium, 400 mg of vitamin E, 300 mg. of magnesium, calcium, and Co enzyme Q 10 in a bottle of multiple vitamins. I never took the prescribed beta blocker pills because I was afraid of the side effects of depression, which I didn't have in the first place.

I was an optimist, always full of hope for doing things the natural way. I preferred Yoga, meditation, serenity, good nutrition, and the vitamins and minerals that keep me calm and cool.

Talk to your doctor before you make any changes in what you do because each person is different and reacts differently. It's in your individual genetic reaction, expression and signature.

For me, today, stretching with Yoga also helped my menopausal back aches. And taken with the best nutrition plan for my insulin resistance, Yoga gives me the right kind of weight bearing exercise I need in this decade.

6

How to Ghostwrite Medical or Specialty Marketing Advertorials and Infomercials

What's an advertorial and how do you write one?

An advertorial is an advertisement promoting the interests or opinions of a corporate sponsor, often presented in such a way as to resemble an editorial. See the dictionary definition at: Answers.com on the Web site at: http://www.answers.com/topic/advertorial.

Medical journalists can write advertorials for flat fees. As a freelance writer/independent contractor you can write medical or other advertorials for various media groups and organizations. To write a medical advertorial, stay totally objective, and tell the truth.

Be practical, honest, and forthright. Include pitfalls to avoid and use insight, hindsight, and foresight. Practice writing editorials in the style of newspaper and magazine editorials you read in most medical magazines and healthcare or fitness magazines going to consumers as well as editorials in trade journals going to people who work in a certain industry.

Writers who write editorials and advertorials still have to sell the product with words. You need to be both convincing and touching without crossing a barrier that separates the emotional gut response from the practical, rational reality.

To the extent that you will be selling the product in the advertorial, keep separate files on all your advertorial sources and resources. Don't mix your advertorial sources with the research you'll use for other writing such as features and news articles. When writing an advertorial, you will be selling a product by building around the product current news and editorial writing. Sometimes an advertorial will be presented as a feature article.

Stay away from advertising sales. Don't ask for any type of commission or cut from the sale of the product about which you write in the advertorial. When you write advertorial copy, negotiate your contract so that you are free from involvement in sales of the product or commissions. Most likely, you'll get a byline, or your name will come up in the future linked to the product. Stay clean of any involvement in the sale, and focus on writing truthful copy.

Negotiate only with public relations officials, not with the advertising agency's clients. If your advertorial, for example, is for a new food supplement, don't deal directly with the manufacturer of the supplement who hired the advertising agency. Work with the public relations people, the marketing communications managers or public relations director.

That way, you are clean of connections, commissions, sales, or kick-backs from the company that makes the product. The information you receive should come from the public relations director.

Fair and accurate writing is what advertorials are about. When you write an advertorial, hand in a regular type of article on the topic you're assigned. The article will be about the product or a medical or healthcare-related subject.

Slant the article toward positive results and problems solved. You'll have a public relations person supervising your work to look at special sections. You may have to cut out some of the references to non-advertisers. So focus on the advertisers in the one and a half page space you're allowed. Each advertorial runs approximately 450 words each.

The current flat-free rate is about $300 per advertorial. This is work-for-hire and usually is copyrighted by the organization that hires you to write advertorials.

Work for hire differs from assigned freelance articles where you supply the idea first and write a query letter asking for a go ahead to proceed and write the article. With work for hire, the media group tells you in advance where the advertorial will be published and contracts with you for a flat fee and the copyright on the advertorial.

The advertorials you write appear in major consumer and women's interest magazines. Advertorials take about three hours to write on average. You'll earn up to $100 an hour, which comes out to about $300 flat fee for each advertorial. As a freelance medical writer, you'll be writing advertorials about subjects that you'll also write journalistic pieces.

What about ethics? People that you interview may become angry with you when they see their quotes and comments published on an advertorial section of a publication. Prepare people you interview for this. Let them know you intend to use their quotes both in the advertorial section and in future feature articles you may write on the subject of their expertise or experience.

You can explain that the part of the magazine in which they'll be featured is supported by a company or is part of an advertisement. It's going to be rough when they see their photo, quotes, and comments on a page reading "paid advertisement," unless you've prepared them and gotten their written approval and photo release for the advertorial.

Also get written permission to use the interview in another article in addition to the permission you will get for the copyrighted advertorial where all rights to the company that hired you to write the advertorial. Work with your public relations director. Find out whether a magazine will publish an advertorial only if the client buys an advertisement. All your sources must be informed of where their quotes and comments or photos will be published and who will own the rights to what they say and the use of their photos.

After you interview people and take their photo, if the editor rejects your work, or if your sources are not used, you must explain to your sources why their information was not used. Prepare them in order to make sure there are no surprises. Otherwise, they might go over your head to your public relations director or to the ad agency's client to complain about the writer. It's impossible to please everyone, but it is customary to inform people you've talked to whether their information will be used or not and explain why.

How to Write an Advertorial for a Medical Publication

The purpose of an advertorial is to inform, not to direct. Collect as many quotes as you can get for your advertorial. The quotes need to come from credible, reliable people and experts that have experience with the product. They are your bread and butter. Outline your advertorial to be a news story, even if it is supposed to look like an editorial. Pare the excess words down to only what you need—bare bones. Include information that will hook the reader's attention right up front in the first sentence and paragraph. The advertorial should never look like an advertisement, but you and the reader knows it is an advertisement.

Be excruciatingly specific. Don't generalize. Support each sentence with reference to a study with dates and sources so the reader can check out the information for credibility.

In only 450 words, you can't use words that aren't crucial. Interview the advertiser for facts, but don't make any kick-back deals. Use the facts after you've checked them out yourself for credibility and reliability. Call the owner of the corporation or the manager. Keep asking to speak to representatives so that you'll have important, valuable facts for your advertorial.

If the medical product is something sold retail, talk to retailers for quotes, especially if you're writing for a trade journal. For general consumer magazines, talk to experts in healthcare and people who have used the product.

Don't use boring specification sheets because the public will avoid reading dull facts in a general consumer magazine. Instead, use quotes. Use those quotes in bold to impact the reader and hold attention. You get less than 20 seconds of a reader's time on an advertorial that's about a page and a half in length—those vital 450 words. An advertorial is more like a 110-word audio book review than a newspaper editorial.

Use quotes in larger type when certain phrases come right to the point that you want to make. Start by reading the literature published by the advertiser. Ask the manufacturer and the public relations director with whom you're working what he or she wants readers to learn and understand by reading the advertorial. Find out what specifics the manufacturer wants you to emphasize. What do they want the readers to understand? Interview each advertiser.

As an independent contractor, you find out from your public relations director or media group what day the publication will run your advertorial. Ask who reserves the space—you or someone on the staff of the public relations or advertising agency hired by the manufacturer or advertiser.

Keep your deadline visible. Ask how much space will be given and how many words they want you to write. With consumer magazines, advertorials are paid for in the same manner as regular advertisements plus the writer's flat fee, which you can bill at about $300.

Generally from the time you sit down at your keyboard with an outline or plan and your quotes, it takes about three hours to write and revise an advertorial. Figure anything up to $100 an hour is fair.

Stay organized. Practice writing advertorials for your own items or freelance articles written that you'd like to market or for your own author's biography. Put your sample advertorials on non-existent sample products on your Web site to advertise your ability to write advertorials. Use mock-up samples for practice. Use specific information on your Web site to sell your advertorial writing skills as you would sell a mock-up magazine. Combine your sample advertorials with an informative column. You can also write infomercials, which are 28-minute scripts for cable and satellite TV stations or for exhibits, expos, and trade show VCRs and DVDs.

How to Write Medical Infomercials and Netfomercials

Write infomercials and netfomercials for trade shows, expos, conventions, training, or cable and satellite TV stations or instructional video/DVD. Here's how to start. Infomercials generally are presented on television or played at trade shows. Netfomercials are presented on Web sites on the Internet.

The National Infomercial Marketing Association

As a condition of the National Infomercial Marketing Association (NIMA) membership, guidelines on refunds, guarantees, warranties, and prices are required. Not all infomercial producers are members of NIMA. Not all clients of infomercial producers are members either.

It's the client who makes the product, then hires an infomercial producer as an independent contractor or freelancer. The infomercial producer either hires a freelance infomercial video scriptwriter for the project or has staff writers working in-house. Some video producers specialize only in making infomercials and nothing else in a local area.

Among NIMA members, if a guideline is violated, a complaint is presented to a review board—two NIMA members and three consultants. If the board finds a violation, the program must be removed from the airwaves within 10 days.

Members in good standing can certify TV station and cable networks that each infomercial complies with the guidelines. NIMA provides telecasters with a list of members in good standing every six months. By codifying the conduct of infomercial producers, the infomercial industry can be lead out of a difficult period when many viewer's attitudes toward infomercials were low.

Regulations set by NIMA state in part that each video will be preceded and followed with a clear announcement that it's a paid advertisement. There must be sufficient product to meet the demand within 30 days. There must be reliable evidence for all claims. Testimonials from consumers have to be voluntary and from bona fide users of the product. The stated price of the product must disclose all additional costs, postage, and handling.

Writing Medical/Health/Fitness/Nutrition Video News and Publicity Releases: A Home-based Business For Freelance Writers

Description of Business:

Send video news releases (VNRs). Produce video public relations presentations on tape for the media and for other clients and corporations. Send video publicity to video customer leads. Use a frequent video buyers mailing list.

Promote author's books on videotape by the following methods:

A. Throw video book parties.

B. Visit local bookstores and libraries to show your video on local author's books and have them come into the store or library for book signing sessions or short talks to follow the videos. Authors who live out of town and who can't afford book tours, can send themselves on tour via your traveling book promotion videos—to anywhere in the world.

C. Compile a list of book reviewers and send them your videos which contain interviews of several authors and their books on one tape.

D. Keep a list of retailers, niche bookstores specializing in the subject of various author's books on videotape, such as new age bookstores, cookbook stores, or mystery bookstores.

E. Visit schools with your videos and market or rent to teachers to show their classes your authors and their book excerpts or promotional trailers on video.

F. Produce instructional aids on videotape to promote a variety of author's works as well as your own videos.

G. Network at professional organizations. Volunteer to be on panels at conventions or conferences, and link up with associations who can promote your videos or video work.

H. Go to as many events as you can where the subject or theme is similar to what you have on videotape. Video people also belong at national bookseller's conventions to promote the authors on their tapes to the press or book buyers. You'll gain visibility to among video buyers.

I. Write articles about how you made your video or where you get your ideas, and send them to any publication interested in reviewing videos, book reviews on video, authors discussing their books or being interviewed on how they get their ideas. Interview others on your niche subject about where they get their ideas from and put their responses on video.

Produce video fireside chats with famous people or authors to promote them and yourself. Nothing promotes your first video as much as your second video (with a free advertisement or trailer in your second video about your first).

Seek out special audiences through their trade, cultural, or professional associations. Video press releases on tape go to the broadcast media and video press as well as the interactive multimedia press. Your mission is to use your video camera to create visibility through the power of the video press—for your business clients, individuals, and yourself. You send a video press release to create credibility as well as visibility.

Income Potential for Ghostwriters and Byline Writers

Charge approximately $200 for a video press release of each client equal to about two pages (two minutes) of a narrated script. You will be able to include ten to fifteen press releases on a-30-minute video tape. A thirty minute tape of only one client is called an infomercial.

Short, two-minute "bites" of many clients on one tape are press releases or video trailers designed to create visibility, identity, and credibility for your client's business or statement to the broadcast/video press. Charge about $100 per minute for your press release services and other video publicity. The amount you can charge varies with your location and reputation and the budget of your clients.

Charge clients a fee, usually $100 to $200 a minute to get on your tape. You can have up to 30 clients on a 60-minute tape all advertising what they have to sell—and you can use direct mail marketing to mail the tapes to people's homes or businesses from a mailing list that focuses on the kind of customer you want. Mailing lists are available by demography, age, interest, profession, or other characteristics.

If you're commissioned to write a script and a feature article, the current rate is $600 to $800 per two-thousand to three-thousand word feature article, plus mailing expenses. Longer scripts are usually about 10-12 minutes. You can bill at $200 per minute for a longer script.

Written contracts are necessary. Ask for one half of the payment in advance, and the other half upon completion. The contract should stipulate that you are to be paid for labor even if the video or feature article is not produced or published by the media.

Charge a monthly $50 retainer for public relations services to clients who can afford to keep you "retained." Expect an hourly fee of $25 for writing video script press releases or print press features and releases.

An additional $50 to $75 an hour fee may be charged for producing, editing, and distributing your client's video to your targeted audience. If you're doing only taping with a video camera, the current rate is $75 an hour for taping only.

Best Locale to Operate the Business:

In big cities like New York or Los Angeles, you'll have competition from the large public relations agencies as well as the video firms preparing press kits for the broadcast media. So you can safely work in any location you choose. Medium cities are best to begin.

Training Required:

It's good to have a course in public relations and a course in video production, but if you read enough books on these two subjects, you can at least get started. See the list of books recommended at the end of the section titled, "Related Video Opportunities." It's a good idea to consult the video trade publications as a way of training yourself to be a video publicist (broadcast and electronic public relations consultant), video press release producer, or video advertising consultant.

Video trade publications provide listings of television, commercial, and industrial producers, sound recording studios, editing and post-production facilities, music/media libraries, casting directors, unions, guilds, and agents. Specialties such as educational videos, public service announcement, and training films are listed. They are good sources to find the information you need about running a video-centered public relations service.

In public relations, the training you learn by yourself, hands-on the job is the best way to learn about the field. It's also a good idea to read several books on how to write press releases and how to run a small, home-based public relations agency. You can find such a list under "public relations" in any college library.

General Aptitude or Experience:

The best aptitude is to have "antennae" out for all possible sources and resources in your environment that can create credibility and visibility for your client and provide free publicity, especially on video tape. Learn how to write a press release, which is the format used to inform the media or client of the news worthiness of a business, person, service, or event.

Video Equipment Needed:

You'll need a video camera, editing equipment, tape, two VCRs for playback and duplicating tapes, a computer and printer (or typewriter) for writing the press release as a script, and the use of a teleprompter so your narrator can read the press release on video tape. You'll also need a device for writing titles on video-tape—which you can do from your computer with video title-writing multimedia software.

Operating Your Business:

Write your press release in script form. It should be two pages long or less—less is better. Each page of script equals about one minute of video time. If you need instruction in how to write for the video market, see my book, 175 Ways To Make Money Writing For The Video Market. A sample video script format one-page (one minute) video press release also appears at the end of this book. Use it as a guideline.

Two dates should appear at the top of your script: the current date and the date the video press release should be released. You can also write "For Immediate Release" on the video label.

The written script should accompany the video script if it's going to the broadcast press. Many press releases will be put on one tape. A thirty minute tape usually holds 15 two-minute press releases. Some press releases may only be one minute long, such as a public service announcement, or a press release to sell a book by video publicity.

Put a catchy title or headline on your video press release. Include the written version of each press release with the video. List the titles on the label in the order that they appear on tape. The name and phone number of the person to contact should be included in a print press release sent to accompany the video press release. If the tape is going to television producers, include the names of the persons on the video in case a producer wants to "book" your client for an interview or to appear on a television talk show or radio program.

The written version of your press release is always doubled spaced and under two pages long. The script version doesn't have to accompany the video, but the written press release does because it describes what's on the video.

Begin writing the press release with the name of the city where the video was made in capital letters. The press release should describe clearly what's on the video—facts like who, what, where, why, when, and how.

The key on video content is to keep asking why the broadcast media will care enough about your video press release to air it as newsworthy. What's your point of view? If the video fascinates, it will sell. You don't want it to be obvious that you're trying to promote a business. Producers know that already. Make the video less promotion and more fascination—with a great visual news angle for broadcast. Send shock waves and startling statistics through the air, but make it appropriate for family viewing.

A written press release uses third person, not first. A video press release can use either for impact. Use a variety of quotes and cuts in the video—like a miniature infomercial without be obviously commercial. Keep in mind there has to be a news angle.

In your written version, at the end of each page, type "more" so editors will know, and type three asterisks *** at the end of the story. In your video version, quick cuts and montages, that is, a series of cuts and images can convey a shift or the end. Use facts, frameworks, and concepts to form an umbrella from which your video press release can hang together with smooth transitions between cuts.

To submit your video press release, call the producer of your targeted television shows. Get the spelling of the producer's name on your mailing label. If you need a directory of media information, get a copy of *Beacon's Publicity Checker.* See the Web site headlined, "How To Be Your Own PR Agent & Save A Bundle!" at: http://www.tulenko.com/SuccessTips/N-08.html. Consult the various Media Directories. The directories are in most main public or university libraries. Editions are published in different categories—for radio, T.V., or periodicals.

Before you mail your video press release or any other public relations features on your client, call the executive producer of the television or cable station you target. Find out whether the producer is interested in the subject of your client's specialty.

Instead of selling your client's book, product, personality, service, research report, survey, or news statement, instead ask the producer what kind of information he or she wants at this time. Always follow up your video press releases to see whether the producer has had time to look or has at least received your video package or press kit.

A press kit contains a video, written press release, feature article, and a photo of the person on tape with a brief biography. The radio market gets the same press release with an audio tape. The print media gets only print information and a photo.

Follow up with a third call to ask whether your video is going to be used. If you want your tape back, enclose a self-addressed stamped envelope large enough to hold the tape.

Your video will be used only if it's timely. The news angle or newsworthiness doesn't count if the news is already old. Send one video press release each month and a print press release once every two months as a follow up. Producers do have a high turnover rate in television. If one rejects it today, next month it may be news.

Keep your eyes open to the various newspapers and other publications to find subjects for video press releases. Video press releases in demand include good business surveys and trend forecasting, business predictions backed by sound science and economics from professionals with credentials and experience,-life-style forecasting and trends, studies of differences between men and women—such as abilities, the job outlook, human interest stories that apply to everybody, and health news.

Pepper the video with the best quotes you can find. Keep the video factual so that anything said can be checked out. The news angle on video must be creative, more creative than the average print press release—and creditable.

Print press releases usually fall into the category of new business openings, new products, awards, benefits to the public, and the results of how new scientific studies impacts the people. Video press releases must reach one octave higher in that they need to have a visual news angle to make an impact. To be a video public relations consultant, you need to find what's visually interesting about your story.

Target Market:

A video public relations consultant who puts press releases on videocassettes needs to reach producers of cable, television, and non-broadcast sources as well as interactive and multimedia shopping channels. Other markets include other people's video tapes—putting the press releases on as trailers or advertisements at the start of video feature films for home video markets, and on CD-ROM computer disks that incorporate video tape.

You can also target trade shows and exhibits where videos demonstrating products play continuously at conventions. You can send through direct mail marketing your video tape to people's homes directly, using a mailing list purchased from your client's mail order, direct mail, or catalog business. On such a videocassette, you can include 15 other press releases on a 30-minute tape or 30 press releases on a 60-minute video tape. Each person seeking publicity or even paid advertising on your video tape can pay you a fee to get on the tape.

Target new businesses, nonprofit organizations, physicians and scientists with new findings to announce, politicians, and public speakers. Financial planners, ministers, retailers, high-tech corporation chiefs, and pharmaceutical firms tend to be heavy users of free lance video publicists. Mental health professionals, attorneys, and physicians also hire video publicists to help book them on talk shows or to announce breakthroughs or new books.

Related Video Opportunities:

Politicians often ask for campaigning videos to be made before an election. Public relations consulting with a specialization in the video and broadcast media is open to any producer, writer, distributor, direct mail marketing consultant, account executive, or independent contractor. A related field is interactive multimedia and the computer/video game market.

`You can also produce infomercials. Video public relations is closely related to offering classified video advertising on tape. An easy way to start is to list classified ads or personal ads—for singles, perhaps, or to sell recycled household products through a video advertising hot sheet.

Direct Response Television Combined With Publicity Service:

Video public relations is related to direct response television (which is related to producing infomercials). One business specializing in direct response television usually handles marketing strategy, commercial concepts, taping commercials, 800 numbers, data processing, credit cards, shipping and handling, media buying, radio, television, and print advertising, logo creation on video, and public relations services.

For further information, see the <u>Broadcasting/Cable Yearbook</u>, Lawrence B. Taishoff, publisher, Broadcasting Publications, Inc., 1705 DeSales St. NW, Washington, DC 20036. Also consult <u>Burrelle's Media Directory: New York</u>, Burelle's Media Directories, 75 E. Northfield Rd., Livingston, NJ 07039.

You'll need to see <u>CPB Public Broadcasting Directory</u>, Corporation for Public Broadcasting, 1111 16th St. NW, Washington, DC 20036, and the <u>All-In-One Directory</u>, Gebbie Press, Box 1000, New Paltz, NY 12561. Most helpful for locating producers is <u>Back Stage</u>: TV/Film and Tape Production Directory, Back Stage Productions, Dept. EB, 1515 Broadway, NY, NY 10036.

Direct response TV marketers can make extra money by producing and writing infomercials, which are broadcast direct mail marketing ads and audience tracking of television viewers who shop by watching television. Direct mail copy writing and producing for video telemarketing is one of the highest paying freelance writing available.

Writers who specialize in writing direct mail copy for both print mail order and video infomercials headed for cable T.V. can create thriving writing and/or producing businesses catering to telemarketing and mail order copy writing corporate clients or write in-house for firms who do telemarketing.

You have a choice of either writing or producing an infomercial or doing both. An infomercial is a long commercial video, running to a half-hour in length, but usually precisely timed at 28 1/2 minutes. It's created to sell by telemarketing. The best infomercial producers use around 400 cuts with music. Many people are interviewed in the infomercial.

Infomercials wait for audience response. The viewer orders the product or service by phoning a toll-free number or sending money to an address flashed on the screen to order the product.

A demonstration video script that solicits audience response through telemarketing on cable stations, or a videobiography script for non-broadcast television personifies and proves a point. Read the book <u>Response Television</u>, by John Witek, Crain Books, Chicago, IL. (1981), to get an idea of how response television works. Also read <u>Television and Cable Contacts</u>, Larimi Communications Associates, Ltd., 5 W. 37th St., New York, NY 10018 (212) 819-9310.

Income Potential:

Video producers of infomercials charge by the hour plus production expenses. The current fees vary with location and complexity of job required. Some producers charge $35 an hour plus expenses of production. Others create a budget with all expenses first, including cost of tape and crew's requirements, then add an hourly fee, plus the post-production editing and distribution expenses.

Best Locale to Operate the Business:

Infomercials can be produced on-site at any location of a business. Being near your clients helps. Big centers for production of infomercials include Los Angeles, San Francisco, San Diego, New York, Chicago, and Orlando, Florida. San Francisco is the hub for multimedia and interactive infomercials, including the San Jose/Silicon Valley area for the software infomercials.

Training Required:

It's best to take courses in video production or read books on how to produce infomercials before you begin. Join professional associations and volunteer. Attend trade shows for infomercial producers and watch a variety of infomercials. Study the number of cuts in popular infomercials.

General Aptitude or Experience:

Creativity, imagination, and experience with a variety of sales and marketing alternatives are beneficial. You're always offering the benefits and advantages of a product. Therefore, sales and marketing training combined with video production experience or coursework is best. It will save you money if you can write your own scripts as well.

Video Equipment Needed:

You'll need your video camera, narrator, host to do interviewing, editing equipment or access to video editing services, your video crew, and a good sound stage or work area to tape the commercial. There should be an audience, and special effects to show the phone number and address where television viewers can phone or send in the order for the product. You'll need to hire operators who take the call on a 24-hour basis. Charge the phone expenses to your client's budget.

You'll also need a computer to track your customers so you'll have a list of television viewers who shop after watching infomercials. Watch infomercials and note the special effects used.

Operating Your Business:

Escape doesn't work in a how-to infomercial. A viewer watching a tape on on how to buy real estate doesn't want to be swept away to a castle in a fantasy setting for long. It might work in an infomercial selling a general idea or theory that applies to many people in many jobs, such as how to get power and success in relationships or careers.

Infomercial scriptwriters don't resort to gimmicks. They give information for decision-making by presenting the facts in as straightforward a manner as possible for intelligent decision-making. The questions of who, what, how, why, where, and when are answered as in an in-depth straight news article.

The viewers want to be well-informed before they spend their life-savings, their "blood money" on a cable television advertisement. They are wondering whether they can buy it cheaper in a store or at the swap meet as they dial the phone.

Will they be hit with a handling and shipping charge that raises the cost another ten dollars? The customer wonders what happens when they give their credit card number to a total stranger on a toll-free number across the country. Who else will have access to that credit card number?

Some beginning infomercial writers turn out scripts that use the techniques of a Hollywood filmmaker to make people watch. Instead, they should be writing to make people buy one brand over another. There's no correlation between a person liking an infomercial and being sold by it.

Use factual, direct, tough commercials because they work. Hard hitting, informative infomercials and commercials sell a product where the customer is watching solely to get information. Soft-sell imagery doesn't work in infomercials like they do in 30-second commercials selling the imagery of the pleasure of eating a bar of chocolate.

Infomercials emphasize believability, clarity, and simplicity over creativity. Don't write confusion into a script by putting in too much dazzle, sensation, and entertainment that overpower the information and message. The emphasis is on helping the customer make a sensible purchase.

Small budgets often do better than big ones in the infomercial for cable T.V. production. TV's longest-running commercial which offers a record set of "150 Music Masterpieces" through mail order by phoning a toll-free number, was made in 1968 for only $5,000. It sold millions of dollars worth of records through mail order because of this one television advertisement.

There are a dozen types of infomercials. They include the following:

1) Product demonstration.

Scripts are used for trade show exhibition and continuous loop playing.

2) Testimonials.

Real people on tape add credibility for a product.

3) The pitchman.

A straight narrator delivers a sales pitch on the product to give factual information in the shortest period of time. This is a talking head short that should only be used for brief commercials or a scene in an infomercial of less than 10 seconds.

4) Slice-of-life.

This is a dramatization between two people and a product. In an infomercial or training script, the dramatization is a framework that can be used to portray true-life events to teach people how to make decisions or how and where to get information.

5) Socio-economic lifestyle.

The social class of the user is emphasized to show how the product fits into a certain economic class such as blue collar, yuppie, new parent, career woman climbing the ladder, or senior citizen retiree.

Examples are Grey Poupon, the upper-caste mustard selling to social climbers and Miller Beer dedicated to blue collar workers celebrating the idea of the working man and woman being rewarded for hard labor with a cold beer.

6) Animation.

Cartoon infomercials sell to children in school and at home. Adults become impatient watching a cartoon demonstration. Animation is expensive to produce for cable television. Use it only to sell to children or to sell supplies to professional animators in non-broadcast demonstration video tapes used to sell products through mail order or at an animator's trade show or exhibit.

7) Jingles.

Lyrics work in short commercials because they are remembered. A best-selling board game called 'Adverteasements' makes players recall all the advertising jingles and trivia information from their past. Ask any person in the street to sing the jingle of an advertisement, and chances are he or she will remember the jingle.

8) The mini-feature film with visual effects.

(Case studies don't report that action set in fantasy scapes sells more products.)

9) Humor.

In short commercials humor works well as in "Where's the beef?" In long info-mercials, it distracts from the information. Some humor can be used to prove a point in a long commercial. Infomercials sell credibility. Humor distracts from believability.

10) Serial characters.

A fictional character that appears in print ads and short commercials, such as Mr. Whipple or the Pillsbury Doughboy is very effective.

In a longer commercial, viewers will soon tire of the fantasy character and change the channel. Infomercial viewers want to see real people's testimonials, people like themselves with whom they can identify. Keep the fictional character out of a true-story informational commercial. People want references. Give them references who testify why the product works so well.

11. Tell-me-why infomercials.

Give people reasons why the product works as it does and why they should buy it. Copy works better in print than in a short TV or radio commercial. However, in an infomercial for cable, satellite, or trade show use, obtaining "tell me why" information is the reason people watch in the first place. Viewers want the writer to explain why and how the product should be used and what need the item will fulfill what problem it will solve, and what result will be gained. Show benefits and advantages.

12. Feelings, Intuition, and Sensation.

Tug at my guilt-strings. Persuasive infomercials use feelings backed up by logical facts that prove a point about a product. Move the viewer by writing genuine emotional copy. A dramatization showing a person shedding tears of joy that someone has telephoned long distance is persuasive. It makes viewers feel guilty they haven't called their mother in years. Infomercials emphasize demonstrations, testimonials, pitchpersons, and straight-sell formulas.

A little emotion within a dramatization can be very persuasive. Either it will sell the product or evoke guilt and anger in the viewer for not having lived up to expectations. The viewer could have conflicting feelings.

He may not want to call someone he dislikes because of having suffered emotional abuse in that person's presence. A whole slew of nasty or sentimental feelings totally unrelated to selling the product can be unleashed by one emotional scene in a commercial.

The emotional, "tug at my guilt-strings approach" works when selling nostalgia. Emotion persuades people to make more telephone calls, or send more candy and flowers by wire.

Using the emotion strategy in infomercials works well for selling sentiment, communications products, craft and knitting machines, charm bracelets, products for the elderly, or greeting cards. Look at the success of the long-running AT&T commercial, "Reach Out and Touch Someone." Who doesn't remember that command to extravert?

To write an infomercial that sells, first find out the producer's budget. Then deliver a selling message within the budget and time limits. Turn the sound off. Can you still understand what is being sold? Sight and sound works together. Use sound only to explain what the picture is demonstrating.

Keep the pictures simple. Use words to make an impact, the fewer the words, the better. The more complex the graphics, the few the words are used to explain them.

Computer graphics, special effects, and animation are expensive. The stand-up presenter and demonstrator cost much less.

Ninety words can be spoken in 60 seconds. Forty-five words can be crammed into 30 seconds. Many 30 and 60-second commercials contain far less words so the viewer can really get the information. Compare this to the print ad which usually runs 1,500 words in a 30-60 second read.

Sell every second the script is on the airwaves. The first four seconds of an infomercial are the same as the headlines of a print ad. The viewer takes four seconds to decide if he/she will sit through the rest of the infomercial or commercial.

Open the infomercial with a real-life situation. It must hook the viewer in those first four seconds. The music and visuals can add the background. The opening is called the cow-catcher. It's supposed to grab the viewer. After seven minutes, the average attention span wanes quickly.

Use motion to keep attention riveted. Show the syrup pouring, the machines working, the demonstrator moving. Let the viewer hear the whirr of the machine as it moves forward. The sound is more appetizing than the look.

Use titles superimposed over the picture to reinforce a sales point not covered in the narration. The address and phone of the company are always superimposed in addition to the narrator's spoken words. What if the viewers are deaf or blind, can they still read or hear the infomercial? Have titles superimposed on the info-mercial saying "Not available in stores," when applicable.

The market for Spanish language infomercials is skyrocketing in the South-west and in California and Mexico. Bilingual video scriptwriters are in demand. In some of the major cities such as Los Angeles and New York, infomercials in several foreign languages are broadcast on cable television's ethnic and foreign language programming stations or on radio.

Some video magazines to sell products are made in two languages, especially to reach the huge Hispanic market in California and the Southwest. Every infomer-cial repeats the product name and selling point several times. Most viewers aren't paying attention when the infomercial comes on. A repetitive script is necessary in this case. The product name and selling point is repeated at the beginning, middle, and end of the infomercial.

Viewers of infomercials get bored quickly if the presenter isn't somewhat dif-ferent. Use a child who looks five years old, for example, to sell a product emo-tionally. Have an adult present the facts and logic behind the demonstration for credibility.

Show people using the product constantly throughout the infomercial. Prod-uct neglect is the primary reason why infomercials don't sell. Show people dem-onstrating, talking about, and applying the product to many different uses.

Proven techniques in print ads also work in television infomercials, such as color reversals, black background with white letters superimposed over a photo, etc. In infomercials, viewers call or write to order the product. Announce this at the beginning with something like, "Get your pencil and paper ready to take advantage of this one-time offer."

Few people sit down in front of a T.V. set with a notepad. It's entertainment time.The infomercial is an unwanted intrusion that angers a lot of people. Late night infomercials interrupt late night films. People may be grumpy at 3:00 a.m. or 5:00 a.m. when many infomercials are broadcast. Prime-time cable infomer-cials interrupt the entertainment. Give people a chance to get out of bed or away from the graveyard shift desk clerk slot and get paper and pencil.

Use a celebrity to do a voice-over or on-camera narration. Identify the celeb-rity by name and superimposed title. In local retail infomercials, give the direc-tions or address of the store. Short T.V. and radio commercial basic lengths run 10, 30,60, and 120 seconds. Infomercials run 5, and 30 minutes. The 30 minute length actually runs 28 1/2 minutes. Infomercial lengths stop short of 30 minutes or 5 minutes to allow for short commercials to be broadcast before and after the infomercial on cable T.V. stations.

The 10-second commercials identify a product to support another longer commercial. Sometimes two different product companies share one commercial—offering two different products. Mail order advertisers use 2-minute infomercials on T.V. to be convincing, then follow up the campaign on cable T.V. with a longer infomercial to give more complete product demonstration. Cooking shows that demonstrate appliances such as food choppers are popular.

A short T.V. commercial sticks to one main sales point. Only in five to thirty-minute infomercials and in print brochures is there the time to cover all the facts. So the only reason a person watches an infomercial or reads a lengthy sales brochure is to consider the facts.

The video script format for infomercials uses the two-column format. Video (visuals) is typed on the left. Audio (sound, music, speech, and special effects) is typed on the right. The video directors are given in upper and lower case letters. The audio or speaking part is typed in capital letters so the narrator or actor can see the speaking parts stand out for easy reading or memorization.

The visuals show the product demonstration. The narration tells the viewers the unique features and benefits of the product. Don't tell how good it is, tell how it will benefit the viewer. The ending makes the most impact. A play on words can lend humor to the script if it also lends credibility to the product and emphasizes how the customer will save money and get superior merchandise.

If something is more expensive on T.V. than it is when found in the store, sometimes the customer is persuaded by being told he's worth it. The emotional impact hits home by asking, "Don't you think I'm good enough to deserve this product?" It works particularly well on wives who know their husbands are very tight with money and affection.

The customer's attitude toward infomercials is "When someone starts to make money, someone else will appear to take it away." To combat this psychological attitude, infomercial producers focus on "target marketing." It's the idea of having different promotional videos aimed at various segments of the market. Software manufacturers may aim an infomercial campaign at doctors by sending video tapes to hospitals' training departments and another infomercial campaign aimed at lawyers—for the same computer product.

A writer of infomercial scripts uses numerous testimonials, endorsements, and product claims highlighted by music, hundreds of cuts to the product, to users of the product, to satisfied customers amidst a background of special lighting and entertainment to maintain the viewer's attention for the half-hour commercial.

The average adult's attention span for viewing a non-fiction video is only seven minutes. The quality of an infomercial writer's script can be carefully measured by audience tracking to see how many orders for the product come in at any time. A video demonstration tape or video magazine acts as a company brochure to sell a product requiring non-impulse buying. The customer still has to come into a store or send away for the product, such as real estate.

This is the age of product intelligence for video scriptwriters. Consumers demand real information. Information has turned the word 'sell' into a noun as in information becoming "real sell." Infomercials on television advertising became popular when the cost of buying time on cable television became low. Advertisers can afford to run five minute to half-hour commercials on cable.

The video scriptwriter of infomercials needs to give complete information and a sales pitch at the same time. Interactive technologies allow viewers at home or corporate viewers at the office or plant to choose which segments of an infomercial they wish to see instead of flipping through a parts catalogue.

Corporate viewers now use their computer keyboards to order products seen on a video tape linked to their computer through desktop video devices. Desktop video enables viewers to interact with a personal computer at home or in the office and with a video cassette tape played on a home or office VCR player and send out orders through a computer modem to anyone's telephone number, usually, with a toll-free 800 number.

Consumers are hungry for information by which they make decisions. A video writer puts in information and leaves out the jingles and other frills seen on short T.V. broadcast commercials that imprint the brain and wring the emotions.

In one survey, 68 percent of viewers said that short commercials don't give any facts about a product. They only create an image. An infomercial is designed to give facts. It's similar to a product demonstration tape script or an instructional video.

Information alone is not remembered. The viewer will always take images emotionally. A creative writer's tendency to achieve dramatic results by waiving the rules works in short commercials where style and form evoke more emotions than substance.

For example, a black background with white lettering where the white lettering is printed over or with a photo background imprints the brain. People remember a reversed color advertisement better than white background with black letters.

The success rates of infomercials that break the rules are unpredictable. Video copywriters use what works to obtain consistently high sales results. In any bookstore the how-to books dominate and appeal to the mass audience reader. People come in for straight information when they want to make decisions on what to buy or how to build it.

How to Write Scripts For the Videos You Will Produce

Use symbolism and metaphor in your infomercial. A script can visualize the waves of the ocean, flow of a river, or waterfall, or ticking of a clock with the handles speeded up to show the passage of time or evolution of a species. A toy crane truck can recreate an accident to teach decision-making.

Use symbolism and metaphor on camera to re-create the events of your life as they flow, perhaps, by showing the flowing river near a client's hometown. Symbolism creates new meanings in a script. The symbol must be recognizable by the audience and cross-cultural. What works in one culture may be taboo in another. Find out what the taboo colors are for the country the video will go to.

For example, in Saudi Arabia, red is a taboo color. Writing is never shown in red ink. In China certain shades of blue signify death. Exporters who featured blue dishes in China found the products didn't sell because of the shade. Color symbols are important if the tape is headed for export.

In video production, symbolism is used in corporate history videos to show the change of a company's product. It can also show someone age on camera or grow up from childhood. Metaphor compares a person to another object.

In an infomercial (to publicize someone's color consulting franchise whose logo is a rose), show the main character or proprietor to symbolize her logo. She is like a rose and is selling a product that is supposed to remind the viewer of everything a rose symbolizes. The product is like a rose. It's colorful,-sweet-scented, and blooming.

To symbolize this imagery in a video script, cut to the leading character's velvet, black hair and pouting, red lips. Then cut to a bouquet of dark, red roses. Then cut back to the character walking through her home dressed in the same shade of red to form a certain imagery of the soul of Spain or a wild, Irish rose.

Then a quick cut to her business, a color consulting firm, where she's matching the red shades of a lipstick to a client's best colors. Then cut to your logo stationery, a red rose. A final cut to a bouquet of red roses is placed in her arms as she welcomes her new baby home, named Rose. (The client may want the baby to turn into the business logo on camera.)

How Do All These Wire Skeletons Fit Together Like an Umbrella To Produce An Infomercial?

A video script's design is composed of all those foundations—like wire skeletons—and edited together, fitted side by side. You need an umbrella under which your concept will fit. The facts plus the basic foundation becomes the concept.

A creative concept is the sum total of each foundation and each fact combined, edited together, fitted so that the whole video or film flows like one piece of cloth with no seams or hanging threads. Is the script sound-oriented for radio, or audio-text? A visually-oriented script with fewer words is filled with symbolism and metaphor instead of straight facts. Which creative concept does the producer define?

Time is budget. A sound-oriented or verbal script's purpose is to <u>persuade</u>, to inform, to warn, to close a sale, to obtain feedback, or to be remembered. A visually-oriented script is there to entertain, evoke emotions, and imprint the imagery on a viewer's brain which will be recalled later without thinking. It's subliminal.

Verbal-oriented video scripts offer information that enable viewers to make intelligent decisions about a product or service. Subliminals imbedded in an infomercial are never revealed verbally. Infomercials and information videos work on the left-hemisphere of the brain, the logical, analytical, decision-making side that seeks verbal information.

Visual-oriental scripts work on the right hemisphere of the brain that controls emotions and imagery. That's where subliminals are imbedded, and art forms evoke feelings. One day a viewer daydreams about that candy bar shown on television next to the image of a beautiful woman in flowing chiffon making romantic gestures. Who can forget the Nestle's chocolate bar lyric in the background that begins, "Dreams like this..."?

Target Market:

Many writers who specialize in writing direct mail order copy (what many people call third class or "junk mail") also write infomercials and commercials for video or broadcast television. Video and audio tapes are sent by mail order along with print advertising copy and information to customers.

Video newsletters may also be included. Direct mail order copywriters for video or print write advertisements, sales letters, and demonstration video scripts to obtain orders for products such as magazine subscriptions and insurance. A company purchases computer-sorted mailing lists of people in certain geographical, income, professional, ethnic, or age groups.

The demonstration tapes or video newsletters are sent to potential customers to motivate viewers to buy a product by direct mail order. An audience-tracking study is followed up to measure the effectiveness of the written copy or the video script. If many products sold through mail order, the writer is judged excellent. The writer's income goes up. The freelancer is now in demand by infomercial producers and direct mail order copy publishers.

Anyone watching an infomercial is an information seeker. A sales video, like a feature film, informs as well as sells escape. The reason to write a nonfiction video script is to create grounds for a decision from the viewer's end. A decision is made not only about a product or service, but about those who identify with the product or feel repelled by the tape.

The infomercial producers set their own guidelines to battle poor public perception of the long-form commercials. The National Infomercial Marketing Association (NIMA) requires members to produce programs based on truthful information in compliance with laws and regulations. Guidelines cover crucial issues such as sponsorship identification, program production, product claim substantiation, testimonials and endorsements.

The National Infomercial Marketing Association's guidelines for members include ordering guidelines. Writers need to work into the script the ways in which customers can order and pay for the product. What prices are fair? Can the customer buy it cheaper in a discount chain? Then why would he order from cable T.V. and pay more? Is it sold in the stores? Are similar and competing products sold in stores, but this product is sold only on TV?

The writer must write copy to sell at the client's prices, sometimes knowing in advance that the customer can get it cheaper in the store than by ordering from T.V. Also, what warranties are on the product? What guarantees do the claims make on T.V.? What are the guidelines for refunds?

◆   ◆   ◆

Writing Popular Inspirational Articles for Health, Fitness, Self-Help and Nutrition Magazines

It makes no difference what religion or spirituality essence you select, but writing an inspirational article or true life experience for the health/fitness/medical, self-help or nutrition publications is in demand and expanding its need for sharing how you solved a problem, obtained results, and received benefits. This type of writing can be in the form of books, true stories, advertorials, scripts, or in featured articles and columns.

What the medical publications and religious or inspirational markets are looking for is sharing commitment, values, and most of all—what you've learned from your mistakes or experiences. Show how you arrived at your choices, and how you've grown and were transformed, gaining wisdom that everyone can share.

By sharing your experiences and life story, readers will learn how you made decisions and why, what wisdom you gained from your growth or transformation, and what made it possible for you to grow and change and become a stronger and better person. The stories you'd write about would be those universal messages we all go through, such as rites of passage, dealing with the stages of life in new ways, finding alternatives, and how you handled the challenges.

The religious and spiritual or inspirational markets want stories that show intimate glimpses—pictures (or visual and visceral words) and **choices.** Show how you solved your problems. Supply the specific examples and facts. The reason people read your story is to find out how to solve their own problems and make decisions. Give them information they can use to make decisions, even if you write fiction. Have some authority and truth in the fiction, particularly about facts and historical information.

People buy your story to make choices, including choices in the later stages of life or choices in growing up and making transitions. As people move from one career to another or from one stage of life to the next, they want to read about how you made that passage in time and space, and what choices you made.

Life story writing should be more preventive than reactive. Biography writing is reactive because it responds only when people are in need, in transition, or in turmoil. What sells is preventive story writing. Give transformation, growth, and problem solving information so people will be able to prevent making your past mistakes.

Show them how you've learned from your mistakes and pass on your wisdom, growth, and change. Readers want to share your understanding. Put rewards and possibilities for personal growth into your life story. Don't merely dump your pain and prior abuse on readers or your history of how you were tortured. That's not going to solve their problems. What will is writing about how you've worked at understanding challenges. Look at your readers as your future selves.

Approach life story writing as you would approach writing song lyrics. Pick an industry and focus on the industry as you develop a life story built around an industry or event. If you write about your own life story, do interviews.

Get many-sided views by interviewing several people you know. You'll discover blind spots you would never have noticed about yourself. Treat your life story not only as a diary with a one-sided view, but as a biography. Interview many people who have had contact with you as you grew up or during the experience you're targeting.

Writing the Forward

If you write a biography of another person as a book, story or article, or as fiction in a novel, you'll need a foreword. This is what you're doing as you first meet the person you're interviewing. Have two tape recorders going at the same time in case one isn't working properly. Get permission to record. Write what you're doing as you first meet the person you're interviewing. It should be about 16 double-spaced pages or 8 printed pages, or less.

Writing the Preface

What is the person most conscious of? What is the individual whose biography you're writing doing right now as you first interview that person? What's the biography going to zoom in on? Describe the body language. In Andrew Morton's *Monica's Story*, Monica stifles a yawn and pulls on black leggings as the preface opens with the title "Betrayal at Pentagon City." The preface summarizes the most important event in the entire biography. It should be about 10 double-spaced pages or 5 printed pages. Is your character going to be the right person at the right time in the wrong place? Or the wrong person at the wrong time in the right place?

Start with the Most Important Action

If you're writing your own experience for a health and fitness or self-help magazine (or a nonfiction book) start with the main character (or yourself) immediately becoming involved in the action if he is or you are not well-known. If your main character is in the news and a known celebrity or royalty, start with the date and season. It's all right to begin with the birth of your biographical character if the childhood has some relationship to the biography. You can describe the parents of the character if their relationship has a bearing on the life of the main character you're portraying.

The less famous or news-worthy your character, the more you need to start with the character involved in the middle of the action or crisis, the most important event. Avoid any scenes where the book or story opens and the character is in transit flying to some destination. Start after the arrival, when the action pace is fast and eventful.

Characters

You can make a great career writing true story medical experience books about people in the news, celebrities, and the famous. If these are the type of books you want to write, focus on the character's difficult childhood if it's important to the story and the character is famous or in the news frequently. To create the tension, get into any betrayals by the third chapter. Show how your character's trusting nature snared the individual in a treacherous web, if that's in your story. If not, highlight your main crisis here in the third chapter.

By the fourth chapter, show the gauntlet or inquiry your character is going through. How did it affect your character and the person's family? How will it haunt your character? Where will your character go from here? What are the person's plans?

Focus on an industry or career, whether it be the world of modern art or computers to get the inside story of the people and the industry and how they react and interact. What is your character's dream? How does your character realize his or her dream?

How does the person achieve goals in the wake of the event, scandal, or other true story happening? Take your reader beyond the headlines and sound bits. Discover your character in your story and show how readers also can understand the person whose life story you're writing. It makes no difference if it's your own or another's.

You may want to bring out your story's texture more by adding a pet character and focusing also on the pet's reactions to your characters. Don't forget the religious markets for medical, true experience, and self-help articles.

7

Writing about Gene Hunters

How Ghostwriters and Journalists Can Empower Consumers with Knowledge about Gene Hunters by Using Plain Language

Empower the general consumer with knowledge about DNA testing for predisposition to diseases or for deep maternal and paternal ancestry when written records are absent. At home-genetic testing needs watchdogs, Web sites, and guidebooks to interpret test results in plain language for those with no science background. Online, you'll find genetic tests for ancestry or for familial (genetic, inherited) disease risks.

What helpful suggestions do general consumers with no science background need to consider? What's new in medical marketing is genetic testing online for *predisposition* to diseases—such as breast cancer or blood conditions. Kits usually are sent directly to the consumer who returns a mouthwash or swab DNA sample by mail.

What type of training do healthcare teams need in order to interpret the results of these tests to consumers? Once you receive the results of online genetic testing kits, how do you interpret it? If your personal physician isn't yet trained to interpret the results of online genetic tests, how can you find a healthcare professional that is trained?

If you're more interested in genetic testing for ancestry, do you go to a genealogist or to a geneticist to interpret the results? What if your interest is in genetic testing for disease risks? Do you go to a physician, a nutritionist, a genetics counselor, or a geneticist to find out how certain foods, medicines, dosages, or other products affect your individual genetic expression?

Online firms increasingly market tests that reveal predisposition to diseases. They show risk rather than a sentence that you'll get the disease. Some of these genetic tests offered online show predisposition to breast cancer, blood clotting, or other genetic tendencies. Each day, there's another genetic discovery ranging from varying the dosages of medicines according to one's ethnicity or race mixture to examining the effects of certain foods on certain peoples based on genetic test results. One example would be lactose intolerance—inability to digest milk without symptoms.

Since the human genome code was cracked in the year 2000, scientists have been publishing the results of genetic research, including maps of human, animal, and plant genes. Genetic tests are easy to take. You rub a felt or cotton swab around inside of your mouth and mail it to the testing company according to directions. Your results can be read online. How do you interpret those results?

If you take the results to your doctor, and your physician has never been trained to interpret the results in plain language, you'll need some guidance on how to choose a physician or genetics counselor who has the current training. If the results also were interpreted online, you wouldn't need to visit your physician to get the big picture.

So when you take your test, and see your results online, write to your company asking them to also put online samples of how results are interpreted. Your individual genes will be different from someone else's, but at least you will be able to see in plain language how someone else's tests were interpreted. So far, no detailed interpretations of tests for disease of anonymous individuals are specifically put online for the consumer with little or no science background. Will this day be soon arriving?

What's certain is that DNA tests for predisposition to diseases are affordable and not expensive. Your genetic test results that you take from online testing firms are **not** put into your permanent medical records. That way, private information won't get into the hands of anyone who requests your medical records, like insurance companies and employers chomping at the bit to find out to what you're predisposed.

I like the online approach because it validates your family history. Predictive medicine is the cure of the future. There is a high demand for breast cancer genetic tests through online testing kits. Predictive medicine is growing rapidly in revenue and in consumer demand.

If you want to find out what a company's revenues are, begin your research by looking at any company's regulatory filings. Under the banner "predictive medicine," you can start your search as a consumer. What sells the most? So far, breast cancer genetic tests are popular.

Look for a genetic testing company online that employs its own physicians and genetics counselors who are trained to interpret in plain language to consumers with no science background on how to interpret the results of the specific the types of tests offered. Look for companies that work with doctor's orders and signed informed consent documents for each test.

What you need before you start your research as a consumer of predictive medicine is to be able to reach professionals online. You may even live or work in an area where it's hard to find a doctor. You need to be able to see your results online and be able to reach someone who can interpret those results in plain language so you can follow the diet, dosage, or lifestyle that best suits your individual genetic expression.

It's all about expertise in interpreting the results DNA or other genetic marker tests. Who has the expertise, and how do general consumers find that expert online? With so few genetic counselors available who are trained (approximately 2,000) how will a genetic counselor explain the results of a genetic test to see how your body responds to various medicine dosages when that counselor is trained to talk about pregnancy?

Using Plain Language, Write about Why Studies of Various Ethnic Genes are Performed

Read the many popular science and national magazine articles about studies of particular ethnic genes. Explain and discuss why the studies are being done, what the results are, and how the findings can be applied in a practical way to help readers from the general population. Here's but one example of how studies on Finnish genes are explained in plain language in popular science and consumer magazines.

Finnish Genes

Check out the Discover magazine article, *Finland's Fascinating Genes, Learning Series: Genes, Race, and Medicine [Part 2]*, According to the article, "The people in this land of lakes and forests are so alike that scientists can filter out the genes that contribute to heart disease, diabetes, and asthma," by Jeff Wheelwright, DISCOVER Vol. 26 No. 04 | April 2005 | Biology & Medicine.

The UCLA study also might help you learn more about your Finn-American medical heritage. For example, Karelians from Eastern Finland and Karelia are being compared in studies to people from Western Finland to see whether or not there are any genetic predispositions in the Eastern Finns and Karelians compared to the Western Finns. The article notes that Karelians and Eastern Finns with short arms and legs may have genes for different genetic predispositions compared to Western Finns with longer arms and legs, but all this is currently under study. Gene hunters described in the spring 1999 UCLA magazine article at: http://www.magazine.ucla.edu/year1999/spring99_03.html and http://www.magazine.ucla.edu/year1999/spring99_03_02.html state that Leena Peltonen, of the world's foremost geneticists, helped to put Finland on the map as a global powerhouse in genetic research. She hopes to do the same for UCLA.

Finland has a small population, isolation, and less immigration than other European nations. The government kept meticulous tax records. As a result, Finland has medical records on individuals that go back more than three hundred years. With carefully written medical and genealogical records, it's one way to trace familial health and ailments as well as family surnames. According to the UCLA 1999 magazine article, "Finland also has a system of free, high-quality health care in which patients trust their doctors and are highly willing to participate in medical research."

According to the UCLA magazine article, "In the 20 years that she has been studying genetic defects, Peltonen has identified no fewer than 18 genes related to such common disorders as multiple sclerosis and schizophrenia as well as more obscure diseases like AGT, a rare and horrific brain disorder found almost only among children in Finland."

In 1998, Peltonen localized the gene for familial combined hyperlipidemia, or FCHL, in a group of Finnish families. According to the UCLA magazine article, "the condition leads to the early onset of coronary-artery disease, which remains one of the leading causes of death in the industrialized world."

Check out the UCLA Human Genetics Web site at: http://www.genetics.ucla.edu/home/future.htm. Or if you're in the Los Angeles area, you can hear guest speakers presented by the Department of Human Genetics, David Geffen School of Medicine at UCLA. In your own area, go the many free lectures on genetics open to the public and learn what scientists are talking about in the fields of human genetic variation, population structure, or temperature sensation.

How can you (as a general consumer) apply what scientists have learned yesterday to benefit humanity today? For example, Peltonen's findings on FCHL coincided with a study by UCLA geneticist Jake Lusis, who localized the same gene using a mouse model. "The two scientists, who only learned of each other's research when each published a paper in the same issue of Nature Genetics, are now working together," according to the UCLA magazine article of 1999 titled *Gene Hunter*. You'll find the entire article on the Web site at: http://www.magazine.ucla.edu/year1999/spring99_03.html.

Check out this 1999 article as well as the more recent April 2005 issue of *Discover* magazine article which also describes Peltonen's more recent work at UCLA in genetic research and particularly with Finnish genes. You'll find that the Internet's Web can act as a springboard to motivate you as a consumer with no science background to read about what is being done in the evolving field of genetic testing.

If several scientists can collaborate, so can a world of consumers. Your goal would be to find out how to interpret and apply the results of any genetic tests to improve your quality of life and health. You don't need a science degree to move into new areas. Scientists are doing this daily.

Consumers need to observe the proliferation of information available online and in libraries. Federal research and the Human Genome Project have been mapping human genes since 1990. Ever since the human genome code was cracked in 2000, a flood of publications, articles, books, DNA testing companies, DNA testing kits, and DNA-driven genealogy services proliferated. What's offered as a result of testing is information. For every gene hunter, there is or could be a consumer seeking practical applications of such research.

Genetics is about preventive medicine. As a consumer, you've got breadth. Scientists have depth. They are only beginning to collaborate with one another and get the breadth that general consumers always had without much science knowledge. Genetics is a horizontal expression of a vertical desire. The consumer represents the horizontal breadth of knowledge.

The scientist's hierarchy sits amidst the vertical tower of scientific terminology. It's about language and communication as much as it's about science. Consumers want tests interpreted in plain language so they can readily apply the results to change their lifestyle.

Do scientists working in different disciplines really collaborate with one another? They have to now that the consumer is involved in the practical side of genetics—information dissemination. Collaboration means understanding how to interpret your test results and apply the research to what nourishes your body.

Writing about Pregnancy Concerns for Women's Magazines

The jobs for many genetics counselors currently are with firms that work with women that have pregnancy concerns. If you want to research this issue on your own, start with the studies of primary care physicians done by the Center for Disease Control and Prevention.

Focus on the particular studies of primary care physicians' inability to handle the overwhelming demand for genetic testing but only after the genetic tests were advertised in the media. Note that these types of studies are usually restricted to certain parts of the country. Any good university library or medical school library has articles and studies on their shelves, but few consumers take the time to research studies concerning the demand for genetic testing, particular tests marketed online. Medical marketing focuses more on TV and magazine advertising of drugs rather than marketing online genetic testing kits in popular magazines.

Is there a way consumers can catch up with technology? Yes, online, if the online material is perceived and verified as credible. So what can the consumer with no science background do—get involved in public policy and team up with scientists? That's the first step—empowering yourself by learning to interpret complex DNA test results if only for your individual markers.

You'll need a physician trained to interpret genetic test results and a genetics counselor on your team, but you need this type of team consisting of consumer and professional—online together. No doctor is going to handle a flood of demand for genetic test kit interpretation. What can you do? You can offer an online company that does nothing but interpret the results and acts as a middle person connecting consumer and physician. What you can do is start that type of online company provided the better mouse trap, that is, the online company that will interpret DNA tests given by other online companies.

Another position the general consumer can take is to seek to regulate the market. You can open a company that validates the online companies. And if you don't want to open a company, you can research and offer information to consumers and to physicians. What if you are a consumer who only wants a genetic test to find out whether you're predisposed to a specific diseas such as breast cancer? Here's a company that I highly recommend, DNA Direct, located in San Francisco. What I like about this company is that it is online and has assembled a dedicated staff of genetic and medical experts. DNA Direct provides direct-to-consumer personalized genetic testing services that help consumers put their their genes in context with their overall health, lifestyle, and environment.

About DNA Direct

The results of each test are paired with an in-depth Personalized Report that combines an individual's unique test results, lifestyle and health concerns with a practical plan for action. Each report includes scientific research and extensive resources. In addition, customers are encouraged to call or email DNA Direct's genetic experts for further discussion, interpretation and/or resources and information. DNA Direct believes that testing is about empowerment—your body and your health are ultimately your responsibility.

And your genes offer tremendous insight and play a vital role in the personal, medical and lifestyle choices you make.DNA Direct is a privately held company, incorporated in the fall of 2003, located in San Francisco, California. The company is staffed by a group of dedicated individuals and genetic experts committed to building a genetic testing service that empowers health care consumers.

Genetic testing offers information that can help people make informed decisions about medical management and lifestyle choices. In the current healthcare model, not everyone has access to genetic testing for a variety of reasons.

In genetics publishing, this is the era of making the Web pay. DNA-driven ancestry, molecular anthropology, and genealogy-related books reached the general consumer market in 2002. In book publishing, each year is the year of the special interest book. The mid-nineties, particularly 1996, emphasized Internet-related books. The eighties focused on the recovery book. Angel books flooded the stores in the late nineties. The turn of the millennium saw an increase in popular diary novel and true life story memoirs. Currently, the human genome—DNA is big news and big publishing. Online genetic testing with direct-to consumer contact provides an open door to predictive medicine research.

As mandated by medical professional societies, genetic tests must often be ordered by a physician and test results are interpreted by a genetic counselor, geneticist, or specialist. In some states, genetic testing must be accompanied by an in-person genetics evaluation and/or genetic counseling appointment.

This approach is limited by the fact that there are only 1,200 medical geneticists and just over 2,000 genetic counselors in the US, most often based in urban areas. The number and type of genetic tests are growing exponentially, and they provide a unique opportunity for consumers to learn more about their health.

DNA Direct's Solution

DNA Direct provides individuals with access to confidential genetic testing using quality-assured tests from CLIA-certified labs. DNA Direct's Web-based genetic testing service redefines traditional, face-to-face genetic counseling and allows individuals to be proactive in managing their care. **Why test?** People seek genetic testing for a variety of reasons, including medical, social, emotional and financial.

- Knowledge about your genes can help you make better decisions for your health and for your family.

- The results of a test can give you specific information about your unique body—and you could be empowered to take actions that really make changes in your life.

- Your genes combine with other factors to influence your health. To understand what your test results really mean, they need to be interpreted in the context of your overall health, lifestyle, and environment.

- From peace-of-mind to prevention or treatment, genetic information can tailor your healthcare to best suit your needs.

How Testing Works:

DNA Direct's genetic testing services are high quality, confidential and convenient. The company offers genetic tests that are scientifically proven and performed by CLIA-certified labs. As new tests become commercially available, DNA Direct has the ability to evaluate and make them available to consumers. DNA Direct's solution is simple, easy to use and a certified genetic expert is available to answer questions at any point in the decision, testing, results and reporting process (M-F, 9:00 a.m.–5 p.m. PST). Here's how it works:

Step 1: Get Informed

Learn about genetic testing and determine whether a genetic test is right for you. Knowing whether a medical condition has a genetic basis can be the first step in taking action to live a longer, healthier life. The Web site features:

- Information about specific genetic tests

- A Resource Center with information on genetic conditions, basic genetic concepts, and family stories

- "Why Take a Genetic Test?" and other information on testing

Step 2: Purchase a Test Online, Submit a Sample

The test is easy, painless and completely anonymous with DNA Direct's secure ordering process. Once ordered, a test kit is sent to you. Each kit contains:

- A cheek-swab home test kit[1]

- A postage-paid return envelope

- An informed consent form

---

1.   Some tests require a blood sample. For these, DNA Direct provides simple tools to help locate a local clinic affiliate to have a simple, anonymous blood sample taken.

To test, simply swab the inside of your cheeks with the test kit swabs. Then mail them to the lab in the envelope provided. If you have already had genetic testing, DNA Direct's experts can prepare a Personalized Report using existing test results.

Privacy is of the utmost importance. All personal information is and remains private. Within two business days of purchase, you will receive a genetic test kit in a discreet mailer.

Step 3: View Results & Personalized Report

When the lab result is ready (7-10 days after sample is received), you will receive an email with a password-protected link to your Personalized Report. Simply click on the link, and log in using the secure email and password. The report can be printed, referenced later or shared with others, such as a physician.

Genes are only one piece of the health puzzle. A person's history, lifestyle and other factors also play an important role. The Personalized Report is an essential component to putting your genes in context and giving him or her tools and information to make informed choices. All DNA Direct's genetic tests are accompanied by individually tailored Web reports, which interpret test results in the context of these factors, and explain them in plain English. A Personalized Report includes:

- Lab results and an easy-to-understand explanation of the results.

- Suggestions on how to improve your health and reduce your risk.

- What your results mean to your family, how to talk with your family or doctor

- A physician's letter should you wish to consult your doctor

- Links to other resources, further reading and support services.

- Toll-free access to DNA Direct's genetic experts for additional support and education. DNA Direct's certified genetic counselors are available from 9:00 a.m. to 5:00 p.m. PST, Monday-Friday, 1.877.646.0222 or via email at expert@dnadirect.com.

DNA Direct's Commitment to Your Well Being

Genetics is all DNA Direct does. Its dedication means consumers benefit from the latest research and developments in this fast-moving area of science. DNA Direct collects genetic news and scientific updates of interest to our customers.

The DNA Direct Web site offers information on basic genetics, diseases and conditions, FAQs, the latest research, and more.

DNA Direct brings its customers the latest news on their health and genetic concerns, and it encourages them to stay up-to-date on the health news and medical research that's most important to them by subscribing to DNA Direct's News Alerts (no personal information, including email addresses is ever shared). For additional information about DNA Direct, services and support, call 1-877-646-0222.

DNA Direct leverages the Internet to offer personalized genetic tests to help consumers make more informed healthcare choices. DNA Direct's confidential genetic testing offers consumers unparalleled access and insight with personalized reports and genetic expert support.

According to DNA Direct's press release of February 9, 2005, the Internet has clearly become a valued resource for consumers seeking healthcare information. Today, DNA Direct is helping people go one step further by providing individuals with unparalleled access to confidential genetic testing, insight into their personal genetic make-up, expert genetic support and links to resources that can help them lead longer, healthier lives.

As a direct-to-consumer genetic testing company, DNA Direct offers consumers an unprecedented array of genetic tests and pairs each test result with a comprehensive, personalized interpretation. The result is a highly confidential means for people to take a more active role in their health and well being.

"Genetic testing can help us understand who we are and empowers an individual to make informed decisions about health management," says Katherine Rauen, MD, Ph.D, DNA Direct's Medical Director. "With just over 2,000 genetic counselors nationwide and even fewer medical geneticists, most people don't have access to genetic testing. DNA Direct is bridging this gap to provide people with a resource to better understand, evaluate and, if they choose, work with their physicians to better manage their health and healthcare decisions."

"DNA Direct provides access to those genetic tests where knowing about your genes can make a big difference, such as when planning a family, selecting a form of birth control or starting hormone replacement therapy," said Ryan Phelan, Founder and CEO, DNA Direct. "It's important to keep in mind that genes are not the sole factor in determining an individual's destiny-family history, lifestyle and environment all play an integral part."

The results of a genetic test can help confirm or rule out a suspected genetic condition or help determine an individual's risk of developing or passing on a genetic disorder.

- Studies estimate that 60,000 to 200,000 people die each year from blood clots. At the high end, this disease kills more people than breast cancer, car accidents and AIDS combined. And 1 in 20 Americans carry a gene, factor V Leiden, which can increase the risk for dangerous blood clots when combined with medical treatments (hormone replacement therapy, birth control pills) or other factors (obesity, smoking, long-haul plane flights). When you know you have genetic propensity for blood clots, you can take action to minimize your risk. (DNA Direct Test at the time this book went to press): Thrombophilia; cost: $380)

- About 35 million people in the U.S.—as many as 1 in 4 people of Irish descent, and 1 in 10 Caucasians—are at risk for a hereditary iron overload disorder that causes a wide variety of symptoms, including chronic fatigue, weakness, joint pain and arthritis. If undetected, iron overload can lead to serious problems, including diabetes, liver and heart disease. But with early detection, effective treatment can stop the progression and even reverse some of the symptoms. (DNA Direct Test: Hemochromatosis; cost at Direct DNA (at the time this book went to press): $199.25)

- About 116 million people worldwide—and up to 1 in 10 Americans—are Alpha-1 carriers. Alpha-1 antitrypsin deficiency is one of the most common genetic disorders worldwide. It is often misdiagnosed, most often as asthma. Early diagnosis can help people at risk take steps to prevent lung and liver disease. A simple genetic test is available for alpha-1 antitrypsin deficiency. (DNA Direct Test: Alpha-1 Antitrypsin Deficiency; cost at Direct DNA (at the time this book went to press): $330).

DNA Direct currently offers the following genetic tests:

- ***Chronic Lung/Liver Disease*** (Alpha1-Antitrypsin)

- ***Cystic Fibrosis (CFTR)***

- ***Hereditary Iron Overload*** (Hemochromatosis, HFE)

- ***Inherited Blood Clotting Disorders*** (Factor V Leiden and Prothrombin)

- ***Infertility Panel*** (Fragile-X, Cystic Fibrosis, Thrombophilia, Hemochromatosis, Chromosome Analysis, Y Chromosome Deletion)

Ask about DNA Direct's tests for inherited cancer susceptibility. All prices include a Personalized Report that **interprets results** and offers personalized suggestions for lowering risk, and making well-informed decisions about healthcare. Each report also includes information about putting together a healthcare team, and how to approach sharing information with family members and your physician. Test prices (at the time this book went to press) start at $199.25. Due to confidentiality considerations, DNA Direct does not process insurance claims but does provide information and documentation should you choose to submit an insurance claim on your own.

About DNA Direct

San Francisco-based DNA Direct is a personalized genetic testing company focused on consumer education, empowerment and support. With a promise of providing "Your Genes in Context," DNA Direct's mission is to empower individuals with insight into their genetic make-up, including risk factors, preventive measures and action-oriented information to reduce personal risk, coupled with one-on-one support from DNA Direct's genetic experts. All of DNA Direct's services are completely confidential. For more information, go to www.dnadirect.com or call 877.646.0222.

Personalized Genetic Tests Offered

The results of a genetic test can help confirm or rule out a suspected genetic condition or help determine an individual's risk of developing or passing on a genetic disorder. Once a genetic condition is known, preventative and/or treatment choices can often be made. All DNA Direct tests are selected to help people make better health care and lifestyle decisions. DNA Direct currently offers the following genetic tests:

- *Chronic Lung/Liver Disease* (Alpha1-Antitrypsin)

- *Cystic Fibrosis (CFTR)*

- *Hereditary Iron Overload* (Hemochromatosis, HFE)

- *Inherited Blood Clotting Disorders* (Factor V Leiden and Prothrombin)

- *Infertility Panel* (Fragile-X, Cystic Fibrosis, Thrombophilia, Hemochromatosis, Chromosome Analysis, Y Chromosome Deletion)

All prices include a Personalized Report that interprets results and offers personalized suggestions for lowering risk, and making well-informed healthcare decisions. Each report also includes information about putting together a health-care team, and sharing information with family members and your physician. Due to confidentiality considerations, DNA Direct does not process insurance claims but does provide information and documentation should individuals choose to submit insurance claims on their own.

TEST: INHERITED BLOOD CLOTTING DISORDERS (THROMBOPHILIA)

More than 19 million Americans carry a gene for thrombophilia. If you are one of them, you can take action to prevent dangerous blood clots and live a healthier life. Studies estimate that 60,000 to 200,000 people die each year from blood clots.

At the high end, this disease kills more people than breast cancer, car accidents and AIDS combined. And 1 in 20 Americans carry the gene, factor V Leiden, which can increase the risk for dangerous blood clots when combined with medical treatments (hormone replacement therapy, birth control pills) or other factors (obesity, smoking, long-haul plane flights). When you know you have genetic propensity for blood clots, you can take action to minimize your risk.

Quality Lab Analysis:	DNA analysis of the two most common mutations in the factor V and prothrombin genes by a CLIA-certified laboratory.
Home Test Kit:	Cheek Swab
Test Process:	Order a test online and receive a test kit in the mail. Use the painless cheek swab in the privacy of your home and mail it to our lab in the postage-paid envelope. When the results are ready, we notify you by email. Log on to your secure, password protected account to get your results and Personalized Report online.
Personalized Report:	Explains test results and interprets your genes in context, considering age, health, lifestyle, family concerns, preventive steps, resources and much more.
Expert Support:	Genetics experts are available to answer questions and provide support (toll-free 877-646-0222 or expert@dnadirect.com)
Price:	$380

TEST: IRON OVERLOAD (HEMOCHROMATOSIS)

Hemochromatosis is an iron overload disorder that can effectively be prevented or treated—but it is often undiagnosed or misdiagnosed. About 35 million people in the U.S.—as many as 1 in 4 people of Irish descent, and 1 in 10 Caucasians—are at risk for a hereditary iron overload disorder that causes a wide variety of symptoms, including chronic fatigue, weakness, joint pain and arthritis. If undetected, iron overload can lead to serious problems, including diabetes, liver and heart disease. But with early detection, effective treatment can stop the progression and even reverse some of the symptoms.

Quality Lab Analysis:	DNA analysis of the two most common mutations in the HFE gene by a CLIA-certified laboratory.
Home Test Kit:	Cheek Swab
Test Process:	Order a test online and receive a test kit in the mail. Use the painless cheek swab in the privacy of your home and mail it to our lab in the postage-paid envelope. When the results are ready, we notify you by email. Log on to your secure, password protected account to get your results and Personalized Report online.
Personalized Report:	Explains test results and interprets your genes in context, considering age, health, lifestyle, family history, preventive steps, resources and much more.
Expert Support:	Genetics experts are available to answer questions and provide support (toll-free 877-646-0222 or expert@dnadirect.com)
Price:	$199.25

TEST: CHRONIC LUNG/LIVER DISEASE (ALPHA1-ANTITRYPSIN)

Alpha-1 antitrypsin deficiency is one of the most common genetic disorders worldwide. It is often misdiagnosed, most often as asthma. In early stages it can cause breathing difficulties, fatigue, and weakness, and eventually it can lead to chronic obstructive lung disease (COPD), emphysema, and liver failure. Early diagnosis can help people at risk take steps to prevent lung and liver disease. About 116 million people worldwide—and up to 1 in 10 Americans—are Alpha-1 carriers.

Quality Lab Analysis:	DNA analysis of the two most common mutations in the Alpha-1 gene by a CLIA-certified laboratory.
Home Test Kit:	Cheek Swab
Test Process:	Order a test online and receive a test kit in the mail. Use the painless cheek swab in the privacy of your home and mail it to our lab in the postage-paid envelope. When the results are ready, we notify you by email. Log on to your secure, password protected account to get your results and Personalized Report online.
Personalized Report:	Explains test results and interprets your genes in context, considering age, health, lifestyle, family history, preventive steps, resources and much more.
Expert Support:	Genetics experts are available to answer questions and provide support (toll-free 877-646-0222 or expert@dnadirect.com)
Price:	$330

PANEL TEST: INFERTILITY

Infertility Panel:

Tests Included:	Fragile-X, Cystic Fibrosis, Thrombophilia, Hemochromatosis, Chromosome Analysis, Y Chromosome Deletion
Home Test Kit:	Blood sample
Test Process:	Order a test online and receive a test kit in the mail. Visit a nearby clinic affiliate to have a simple, anonymous blood sample taken. Mail your informed consent in the postage-paid envelope to DNA Direct. When the results are ready, we notify you by email. Log on to your secure, password protected account to get your results and Personalized Report online.
Personalized Report:	Explains test results and interprets your genes in context, considering age, health, lifestyle, family concerns, preventive steps, resources and much more.

Expert Support:	Genetics experts are available to answer questions and provide support (toll-free 877-646-0222 or expert@dnadirect.com)
Price:	male panel $1248.25, female panel $1,191.50

• Prices subject to change without further notice

Other DNA testing companies online test DNA for ancestry, or molecular anthropology research. Those might be of interest to family historians and genealogists or surname groups seeking a genetic signature of ancestors and descendants related to a common ancestor or particular surname. Some families want to build time capsules that contain not only family history but family medical information for future generations. Some DNA testing companies that are online test for reactions to medicines or foods, such as the speed at which your body metabolizes anaesthetic.

Online you'll find numerous companies marketing various DNA tests or kits. Some of these genetic tests are to find out how your body reacts to various dosages of drugs or even foods and skin products. How do you tailor your medicines, foods, cosmetics, anaesthetics, dosages, or lifestyles to your genetic signature? Can you find out by genetic tests which type of dental anaesthesia you can tolerate and which you're type makes you feel jittery or convulsive? What about tests to find out how your hair tint affects your heart beat? What kinds of tests are out there?

You'll need a consumer's guide to genetic testing kits. Research the various companies online and the studies that include side effects of whatever product or medicine you think you might have to use. Your goal is to safely tailor your environment and lifestyle to your genetic expression or signature.

Consumer's Guide to Genetic Testing

Your DNA, including your ancient ancestry and ethnicity has a lot to do with how your body responds to food, medicine, illness, exercise, and lifestyle, but just how much? And how do you know which DNA kits and gene testing are reliable and recognized?

Learning about DNA to understand and improve your health is now interactive and available to the average consumer, not limited to students and teachers, but to anyone else. In the last few years genealogy buffs, parents, and anyone interested in DNA without a science background took an interest in DNA tests rests that reveal deep maternal and paternal ancestry. Currently consumers with little or no science background are interested in learning about drug metabolism—pharmacogenetics. Referring to the whole human genome that science related to linking pharmacy with genetics is called pharmacogenomics.

How your body metabolizes medicine is as important as how your body metabolizes food. Nutrigenomics is about how your genes respond to food and how to tailor what you eat to your DNA. Consumer DNA interest ranges from forensics and anthropology to nutrition, caregiving, family scrapbooking and healthcare knowledge. Nurses are becoming more interested in DNA.

The DNA consumer revolution began when media broadcasts revealed to the public that fast computers had revealed the human gene code. Once more TV opened doors. Suddenly, a gap between science and consumers had to be bridged by available interactive education.

A proliferation of products relating to DNA emerged. The internet shows DNA summer day camps for students and teachers. DNA testing companies and books emerged geared to the average consumer. Genealogists tried to interpret DNA for ancestry. People left other non-science-related businesses to open up DNA testing companies for ancestry research, contracting out to university research laboratories to do the DNA testing. Again, opportunities opened doors to the public.

Nutrigenomics product marketers sought those who wanted a diet tailored to their genetic signature. Pharmacogenetics reports customized medicines in order to prevent adverse drug reactions. Pharmacogenomics studies the entire genome in relation to chemicals and drugs, whereas pharmacogenetics researches specific genes and markers to look for adverse drug reactions for individual clients or patients. Finally, DNA testing products emerged offering to tailor skin care products such as creams and cosmetics to your individual genetic signature.

If you've had an interest in learning about how to interpret your DNA test results for ancestry, you now can see the links to understanding how to tailor your food, lifestyle, exercise, medicines, supplements, and skin care products—in fact numerous environmental chemicals—to your genetic expression. It's not only about food anymore or ancestry alone, or medicine.

DNA testing also is about kits sent to you directly or to your physician. It's about tailoring to your DNA skin products, cosmetics and anything you put into or on your body that gets absorbed. It's about what chemicals are in your water and home-grown vegetables.

No science background? Don't worry. There's a DNA summer camp near you, or an educational experience in learning about DNA now available to the average consumer. Educators, scientists, and multimedia producers have teamed up to teach you the wonders of DNA, your genes and your lifestyle.

What's left? Physicians and genetic research scientists need to talk more to each other because most family doctors don't have time to read the proliferation of publications reporting new advances in genetics or other areas of science that directly affect consumers. It looks like it's the consumer's job to bring people together through the media and through consumer's watchdog organizations, professional associations, and support groups. Key words: action and public education about DNA through multimedia and consumer involvement. I highly recommend the DNA Interactive Web site at: http://www.dnalc.org/. Consumers need to know more about how to interpret DNA test results for whatever purpose they seek—tailoring diets or drugs, skin care products, or seeking out ancient family history or ancestral lineages. The science is new enough to have many more applications on the horizon that consumers can digest in the future. What can the average consumer with no science background learn about applications of DNA testing currently? Start with the publications and the interactive DNA learning sites.

You'll soon become familiar with the DNA terminology. The goal is to bridge the gap between science and the consumer, let alone the gap between science and medicine. So you'll have to invite your busy family doctor to join you in creating consumer groups. It'll work fine. Doctors and scientists usually are found conversing together at parties.

The triangle now includes the consumer. If you have children, bring them into the fold. There are now wonderful DNA summer camps. So include your children's teachers. Learning about DNA as a consumer might make you wish you had majored in genetics. Link your beginning self-taught DNA studies to your special field of interest such as your healthcare or your ancestry.

For history buffs, there's always molecular genealogy for family history. History buffs can follow population genetics. Anthropology enthusiasts can read about archaeogenetics. Bring archaeology and DNA together.

Nutrigenomics links DNA research to nutrition for the diet-conscious. Pharmacogenetics helps you to tailor specific medicines to your genes. DNA gets into all walks of life and work. Start with population genetics and physical anthropology if you wish. I like the popular book titled: *The Real Eve*, by Stephen Oppenheimer. Carroll & Graf Publishers, NY 2003. Or start with nutrition and genetics. First find out what field you like best—nutrition, pharmacy, genealogy, anthropology, or heathcare—and read a book for beginners on DNA related to understanding your particular area of interest, such as nutrition or family history. It's about discoveries.

- A blizzard of discoveries are published monthly in recognized scientific journals found in local medical school libraries open to the public. Only a few consumers ever look at them, and still fewer physicians. Doctors are busy with so many patients and paperwork or bureaucracy. Consumers may not know information is accessible to them. And few can keep up with the proliferation of material in science publications.

- For information, resources, the research network, and references on pharmacogenetics (education) see the Pharmacogenetics and Pharmacogenomics Knowledge Base Web site at: https://preview.pharmgkb.org/resources/education.jsp. As far as education, the Web site features links and articles on the following subjects: <u>What is Pharmacogenetics?</u> <u>Asthma Case Study</u>, <u>CYP2D6 Case Study</u>, <u>The National Institutes of General Medical Sciences (NIGMS)</u>, <u>Medicines For You</u>, <u>Minority Pharmacogenomics</u>, <u>The Importance of Genetic Variation in Drug Development</u>, <u>Publications</u>, and <u>News Clippings</u>.

- Click on the Dolan DNA Learning Center at: <u>http://www.dnalc.org/</u>. The Dolan DNA Learning Center at Cold Spring Harbor is entirely devoted to public genetics education. The gene almanac is an online resource that provides timely information about genes in education. The Dolan DNA Learning Center is the world's first science museum and educational facility promoting DNA literacy.

- Dolan's Saturday DNA program is designed to offer children, teens and adults the opportunity to perform hands-on DNA experiments and learn about the latest developments in the biological sciences.

- If you're interested in student "DNA Camps" see the Web site at: <u>http://www.dnalc.org/programs/workshops.html</u>. Student summer day camps have fun with DNA and enzymes and study DNA science or genetic biology. Students and high-school teachers can participate. There are a lot of ways to become involved in learning more on these topics. I wish there were DNA day camps for senior citizens newly retired with time free at last, or for parents, children, and teachers to participate and learn together.

The student summer day camp workshops feature such wonderful learning experiences as the genomic biology and PCR workshop. This new workshop is based on lab and computer technology developed at the DNALC in the past year. The workshop focuses on the use of the polymerase chain reaction (PCR) to analyze the genetic complement (genome) of humans and plants. DNA educational centers bridge gaps between scientists and communicators.

Many physicians have not yet been trained in nutritional genomics or in pharmacogenetics—how to correctly interpret a DNA test for consumers. Who advises consumers how to tailor their food or drugs to their genes in ways that consumers can immediately use? Who instructs them how to make time capsules out of their ancestry from DNA reports?

For the time being, it's the bioscience journalist who acts as a communicator, the liaison, the publicist, the broadcaster, the bearer of news, the turner of complex terms into plain language, the reporter and the publisher, showing consumers, physicians, and scientists how to bridge the gap between science and healthcare.

Who acts as the middle person between genetics and medicine or between nutrition and healthcare? Who bridges the gap between the dietician and the geneticist? For now, it's the media, the science writer writing for the mass media or an audience of general readers—consumers like you and I. Who should join the science media team? Check out consumer watchdog groups, concerned physicians, genetics researchers—scientists, DNA testing companies, and bioscience publishers.

Instead of worrying about physician apathy or consumers turning to alternative medicine, let's turn to scientific knowledge available to all consumers if you know where to look and what is accessible. If you want to take charge over how your body responds to food or medicine or lifestyle changes, you need to take control by finding out how your genes respond to what you put into your body from what you eat to the drugs you take to the chemicals in your environment.

Has a local or national newspaper reported on rocket fuel or other specific chemicals in your water supply that went into your home-grown vegetables that made your thyroid go wild, find out what research is being done on the situation. Or if your body responds to various foods in certain ways or various drugs in other ways, you can take control by learning what new advances are available to you. Check out what is credible and what works for you. Minorities may have genes that respond differently to various dosages of medicines. Check out the Web site for research on minority pharmacogenetics at: <http://www.sph.uth.tmc.edu:8057/gdr/default.htm>. The Minority Pharmacogenetics website is devoted to issues of minorities, populations and pharmacogenomics.

Have you ever met a doctor who keeps up with all the latest advances? Who has time? Consumers do. Look at the breakthroughs in the journals published monthly. Why worry that medical discoveries aren't being delivered fast enough to patients or clients if you can see what's happening in the journals?

Consumers need to form watchdog groups and to link up with the media. You need to become involved in accessing scientific pioneers. As a journalist, my job is to convey information to the public to bridge the communication gap. As a consumer, your job is to take care of your body. Nobody should walk in medical or nutritional ignorance when the information you might need "is out there." You don't need any science degree or license to read public information. Let's all bridge the communication gap between consumers, scientists, and physicians.

Consumers want applied knowledge. Here's where to start. On the Web, look at: http://www.nigms.nih.gov/funding/medforyou.html. It's the page for The National Institutes of General Medical Sciences (NIGMS). It's the home page for the National Institute of General Medical Sciences, a component of the National Institutes of Health, the principle biomedical research agency of the United States Government. "NIGMS supports basic biomedical research that is not targeted to specific diseases, but that increases understanding of life processes and lays the foundation for advances in disease diagnosis, treatment, and prevention," according to the Pharmacogenetics and Pharmactogenomics Knowledge Base at: http://www.nigms.nih.gov/funding/medforyou.html.

If your doctor hasn't the time to take advantage of current treatment findings, you as a consumer can read what your physician may not get to read for a while. Picture one future fantastic scenario regarding DNA testing where spouses are chosen based on DNA reports. If this sounds too bizarre, visualize choosing foods based on DNA reports. That sounds credible. The point made here is that you could help to bridge the gap between research and conventional medicine. You and I have our work cut out for us, speaking as a consumer and as a journalist who loves reading scientific articles.

The scene at the "speed dating" table opens with a young woman waving her latest DNA test result under the nose of her blind date. "I'll show you mine, if you'll show me yours," she says, smiling. The fellow opens his DNA test result folder or database. They exchange DNA test result printouts and interpretations. "Hmm...regarding ancestry," he says, "Looks like we're both members of the same mtDNA matrilineal clan."

That could be haplogroup H, L, M, or with whatever worldwide mtDNA haplogroup letter or matrilineal 'clan' they match. "Now let's look at your specific genetic markers and genes tested for adverse reactions to this list of medicines or foods or...." She gazes up at him smiling. "I like your lack of risk for diseases," he says. "And I like the way your gene mutations put you at risk for all these inheritable diseases," she answers.

"Do you also have any inheritable real estate and cash? I'd like to be benefi-ciary." He looks at her askance and holds up a little green bottle. "With this gene equalizer, my risk is greatly lowered." They exchange DNA printouts once more and move to different tables to begin another Dating by DNA interview.

Science fiction version of "blind dating by DNA?" Maybe, but consumers want practical results from DNA testing that they can apply to real-life situations. What kind of personalized medicine can consumers find today regarding genetic testing? How many ways can you use DNA tests? Tailoring your food, customiz-ing your medicines by avoiding adverse drug reactions, looking at your ancient ancestry, family history, or genealogy by DNA through "molecular genetics" and perhaps, choosing your spouse by DNA?

Genetic screening of couples hoping to marry or couples seeking answers to fertility questions have been screened for inheritable diseases in several countries. How many ways can you market DNA tests? For what purposes can you use DNA tests? Who will review the products? What consumers need is a guide to genetic testing kits sold directly to the public or sold only to physicians and healthcare professionals.

Personalized Medicine from DNA Testing Companies

How do consumers or consumer's watchdog groups regulate doctors' services? Are DNA test kits sold to consumers really doctor's services or are they medical devices? Consumers want their healthcare and nutrition tailored to their individ-ual genetic signatures, and they want it to be affordable and available to everyone. The FDA regulates medical devices, not physician's services. Where does a DNA kit sent directly to consumers fit into a definition? Scientists and physicians study haplotypes when they map complex-disease genes. Genetic researchers look at the abundance of single-nucleotide polymorphisms (SNPs). They use terms such as "single-locus analyses."

Consumers want those terms translated into plain language by bioscience communicators, since most scientists and physicians are too busy to continuously write about genes for the public. That's why public education programs about DNA exist, including the summer day camps for students and teachers. We need the training programs and camps also for parents—for entire families from great grandma and pa to elementary school children and teens.

When it comes to studying how your genes respond to food or drugs, scien-tists avoid analyses techniques with limited power and instead focus on economi-cal alternatives to molecular-haplotyping methods. So you, as a consumer, presumably with little or no science background, are in a position to learn about your own genes and about DNA in general.

You can start with some of the DNA public education learning programs open to anyone. Since the gene hunters began to explore the entire human genome, they opened a door to the public for knowledge accessible to all. At first consumers were interested in learning how to interpret their DNA test for ancestry and family history. Next, consumers wanted to know how to tailor their drugs and food to their genes—their genetic expression. Finally, consumers found they could customize skin care products to their DNA reports as well.

Consumers ask important questions. What's waiting for you in a DNA kit that will be valuable to your health? How will you understand and apply the scientific reports to your daily lifestyle? How do you find out whether the various DNA testing companies are credible and recognized by which group? Who are the watchdogs here? Who are the experts? What do you do with the information you receive after a DNA test? Should you test for deep ancestry, adverse response to drugs, or tailoring your food to your DNA? How do you apply the information in a practical way?

Should the consumer only deal with companies that sell their DNA test kits to physicians and similar healthcare professions such as dieticians and genetics counselors? Or should the average consumer buy a DNA testing kit directly from a company that also markets to consumers, bypassing physicians? What do you think as a consumer? Which stance are you taking? For resources and articles, see the Web site at: http://syndromexmenu.tripod.com.

What happens when a DNA testing company sells its DNA tests or kits to companies that turn around and sell personalized nutritional or cosmetics products so that consumers can buy skin products or nutritional supplements customized to their genetic signatures? Is this good for consumers? What do you think? I like DNA testing. The interpretation of the tests is tricky. Results can have a lot more than one interpretation, even for physicians and scientists. So how does the consumer learn to screen the screeners?

Should a company tell consumers which specific genes are tested? Some companies do and others don't. How do you know whether the dose of vitamins you take is beneficial or harmful? Do you need to cut back or add more? What can DNA testing do for you, the consumer, presumably starting with no science background? As a bioscience journalist, I'm not taking sides here, but I really like the variety of DNA tests.

Some types of genetic test kits are sold directly to the public, and others are marketed only to physicians and similar healthcare professionals. From the consumer's point of view, there is always the question of whether the tests are needed and if they are, how accurate and valuable are the tests, and who is trained and experienced enough to interpret the answers?

If you're going to take a DNA test, it could be for ancestry, for nutrition planning, or to see whether any prescribed or over-the-counter drug, chemical, supplement, nutraceutical, food, or herb you take will have adverse effects on your body. For years you could test for allergies to some substances and foods, some chemicals in the environment, but now there's genetic testing.

Specific genes are tested for risk or reaction. The type of consumer most likely to order a genetic test for drug response or a "pharmacogenetic test" would be an individual with medical conditions taking several drugs and concerned how his or her body handled the mix of medicines, food, and lifestyle. Each person has his or her own genetic signature.

You rinse your mouth with a type of mouthwash and send the contents in a small tube to a laboratory, hospital, office, or company to be analyzed. Or you swab the inside of your cheek with a felt tip and send the swab to a hospital or genetic testing company so your DNA—specific genetic markers—can be analyzed.

In a few weeks, you get a report. The genetic testing company looks at specific genes and markers. If you're concerned about drugs, you want to know how slowly your body is breaking down any of the drugs you take or might take in the future. You don't want to gulp down a prescription or over-the-counter drug and have it build up in your body to the point you land in the emergency room of a hospital. The whole point of a genetic test for adverse drug reactions is to alert your physician to adjust the dosage of your medicine or change the type of medicine.

On one side, the consumer sees the physician and scientist diagnosing rare diseases by looking at particular genes. On the other, the consumer wants information on how genes work. Firms that sell gene tests directly to consumers need to fill an education gap. Certain tests can be sold directly to consumers, such as DNA testing for ancestry, genealogy, family, oral history, DNA matches, and surname projects where people with the same or similar last names are matched by DNA to see whether there's a relationship in former times.

What DNA testing companies can do for the consumer is to widely teach the consumer about population genetics—the peopling of the world. How about for disease? Genetic disease specialists have been in charge of this new science. Lately, companies that test DNA now market directly to consumers as well as to their physicians. Here's a chance to educate consumers as well as physicians in everything they need to know about their genes. Physicians want to know how to interpret DNA tests for disease markers. Consumers want this information directly. So there needs to be a level for education for both physician and consumer.

If a DNA testing firm markets directly to the consumer, the test should be interpreted for the consumer and the physician. Consumers are paying to learn what medications to avoid. Allergists usually told people what foods to avoid. What consumers want is to know what foods, vitamins, minerals, supplements, skin creams, herbs, medicines, and other nutraceuticals will work best with their individual genetic signatures. Who will teach them? If the physician has only a few minutes to consult with each patient, who else has the time? Either the DNA testing companies must educate the consumer, or the consumer as an autodidact, must teach himself from reliable sources.

Today anyone with a genealogy hobby an open a DNA testing company and contract out to a laboratory in a university to test DNA for clients. When it comes to test DNA for diseases or drug reactions, it's different than sending a printout regarding the client's ancient general ancestry such as the results of a DNA test for mtDNA (matrilineal ancestry) or Y-chromosome (patrilineal ancestry) in the deep past. Those tests are general and would be of interest to people matching ancestors or learning about population genetics and ancient migrations.

When it comes to tailoring food or drugs to your genotype, how far can DNA testing companies bypass the genetic disease specialists and market directly to the consumer? The answer is as far as it takes to teach the consumer about his or her own genetic expression. When you look for a DNA testing company, ask yourself whether the company diagnoses diseases? Does the company help you choose your medicines, food, or cosmetics according to your genetic signature? Or does the company work with your physician and you. Does the company pass you over entirely and only send the results to your personal physician?

Look at the marketing efforts of the company. Investigate gene research for yourself by the many articles available online and in the medical libraries and popular magazines that go to physicians. If you buy a test, is it affordable? Do you need the particular DNA test?

If one of your relatives has a specific condition you might have inherited that will show symptoms when you reach a certain age or presently, you need to know what you can do to delay or prevent the situation. You need to know that the results of DNA testing are for a particular purpose, such as testing adverse reactions of your body to certain prescription drugs. Find out the value of the tests from reliable sources. If you start with your personal physician, make sure he or she can correctly interpret a genetics test. Some physicians can't because they were never trained to do so.

Consult the various professional associations for referrals to genetic disease specialists rather than rely on a generalist when it comes to interpreting your test while you learn how to interpret your tests yourself. The purpose is to make sure your physician's interpretation and your interpretation agree. If you have any doubt, you need more information and a second opinion.

What you want to avoid is confusion. Are the tests available today reliable? Find out from several opinions of specialists. To reach these specialists, the professional associations for the various genetic disease specialists would be of help as would the publications. You can talk to the research labs at universities specializing in genetic testing. The institutes are online and have their own Web sites.

Talk to federal health officials about what's on the consumer market in your country and in other countries. Some people send their DNA swabs to companies and/or labs in other countries. Currently genetic tests are sold without a special 'watch' organization that reviews them. So look at any publications put out by the U.S. Food and Drug Administration (FDA). The FDA wants consumers to become more involved in their own food safety and security monitoring. Keep a folder on DNA testing company marketing claims and check them out.

Companies can tell you which mix of vitamins works best or what food to eat based on genetic testing and/or health questionnaires. For example, check out GeneLink Inc., New Jersey. Their Web site is at: http://www.bankdna.com/breakthrough_profiling.html.

According to Multex, an investments site at: http://biz.yahoo.com/p/g/gnlk.ob.html, "GeneLink Inc. is a bioscience company that offers the safe collection and preservation of a family's DNA material for later use by the family to identify and potentially prevent inherited diseases. GeneLink has created a new methodology for single nucleotide polymorphisms (SNPs)-based on genetic profiling. The Company plans to license these proprietary assessments to companies that manufacture or market to the nutraceutical, personal care, skin care and weight-loss industries. GeneLink's operations can be divided into two segments, the biosciences business, which includes three SNP-based, proprietary genetic indicator tests, and DNA Banking, which involves the use of its proprietary DNA Collection Kit." Contact GeneLink at: 100 S. Thurlow Street, Margate, NJ 08402. See the Web site at: http://biz.yahoo.com/p/g/gnlk.ob.html.

GeneLink also offers gene testing for skin care products. According to a March 6, 2003 media release posted at GeneLink's "In the News" Web page at: http://www.bankdna.com/news_articles/03_06_03.html,   GeneLink,   Inc.

(OTCBB:GNLK) "entered into a collaborative agreement with DNAPrint Genomics, Inc. (OTCBB:DNAP) whereby the companies will combine certain scientific and intellectual property resources to develop and market "next generation" genetic profile tests to the $100 Billion plus personal care and cosmetics industry. Further details were not disclosed.

"GeneLink invented the first genetically-designed patentable DNA test for customized skin-care products, and DNAPrint brings its ultra-high throughput genotype capability and ADMIXMAP platform to the partnership. The companies anticipate screening millions of candidate markers to broaden proprietary product offerings.

"Tests are designed to assess genetic risks for certain skin and nutritional deficiencies and provide a basis for recommending formulations that have been specifically designed to compensate for these deficiencies."

I like this idea. I'm allergic to hair tint and aloe vera, and it would b wonderful to find skin care products that didn't turn my skin red and make it itch. Think of all the allergy warnings and patch tests on hair products. If everyone walked into a beauty salon with a list of products that can be safely put on the scalp or other skin without an adverse response, that would be my definition of comfort. Also, check out GeneLink's test which tells clients which mix of vitamins is appropriate for an individual's genes without getting an adverse reaction from the vitamin combination. I know certain supplements over-stimulate my thyroid. I'd love to have these kinds of tests.

How about you? Still, you need to do your homework on the usefulness of the tests or the claims. Perhaps you need to deal with a company in another country. Sciona Ltd. in England gives nutritional advice based on your DNA and a questionnaire related to your health. ***The company sells tests only through doctors and dieticians.*** How do you know which defect is associated with any specific gene when the gene is defective? With so many interpretations, consumers can become confused from test results. Sometimes scientists in various companies don't know which results are accurate predictions. That's why consumer watchdog groups are necessary.

The only problem is that the average consumer usually can't afford to hire genetics counselors unless they have a specific genetic disease. If you have a reduced ability to process something, it's not a disease, but unless you take action, your body could suffer in other ways resulting from the reduced ability to process an essential nutrient from your diet that your body needs to work with other processes. It's like a chain reaction.

That's why DNA testing is helpful. At the same time, you can't assume some people need more of one vitamin just because their body processes a nutrient at a reduced rate. The science is still very new. A lot of data is still in the works. You don't know whether certain genetic profiles need special diets. Consumers want to see rare clinical data. Consumers most of all want to know the value of what the DNA tests predict. And no one wants to take a test and then worry for a decade.

What consumers want are not only tests of prescription drugs and food as to whether adverse reactions happen with individuals based on their genetic testing, but personalized anti-aging formulas, cosmetics, creams, and other products customized to the individual's genetic markers are needed.

These tests must be reliable, consumers say. Feedback is helpful. Customer reviews of the companies are needed. Who will publish customer reviews of the products and the DNA testing firms? These consumer reviews could also include input from scientists and physicians. Physicians should take the DNA testing themselves after they are properly trained to interpret the tests before looking at their patient's results.

Nutritionists and dieticians show concern that medical schools only give very brief and shallow courses in nutrition to graduating physicians. What about a course in interpreting genetics tests? Will this be left to naturopaths and homeopaths? Or can medical schools include courses in DNA test interpretation to physicians other than genetic disease specialists? Healthcare consumers should ask for DNA testing from their HMOs before taking prescribed medicines. Will insurance companies pay for testing?

Look at the various DNA testing companies. Also look at health screening companies. One would be HealthcheckUSA, San Antonio, Texas for example, sells a mail-order test for iron buildup in the blood known as hereditary hemochromatosis. Results go to the consumer. If you need a test for cystic fibrosis or a blood clotting disorder known as factor V Leiden, check out this company. Their Web site is at: http://www.healthcheckusa.com/media.html, or you can write to them at: **HealthcheckUSA,** 8700 Crownhill Rd., Suite 110, San Antonio, TX 78209.

Practicing physicians started HealthCheck USA in 1987 to provide health awareness screening to customers throughout the USA. The tests provided to their customers are the same as those ordered by physicians across the country. Many physicians refer their patients to Healthcheck USA. Since 1987, HealthCheck USA has provided over 500,000 health awareness screening tests to satisfied customers nationwide.

The company is associated with the country's major fully accredited medical reference laboratories, to ensure quality, accurate test results. HealthcheckUSA has partnered with <u>Virtual Medical Group, Inc.</u>, to offer physician interpretation of results. According to HealthcheckUSA's Web site, "You can have your results reviewed and interpreted by a <u>Board Certified Physician</u>. By selecting the "Physician Interpretation of Results" option, you will be mailed instructions with the hard copy of your results. These instructions will give you a toll free number along with your username and password to access your interpretation 72 hours after your blood draw. This process is completely confidential, private, and secure."

Here the consumer has the best of both worlds. What tests are provided? Check out the list of tests provided at the Web site: http://www.healthcheckusa.com/testsweoffer.php.

When any company does health screening, find out whether it is DNA testing, blood testing, comprehensive tests, or whether you are sent test kits such as for colon cancer screening, prothrombin (factor KII) DNA test, cystic fibrosis (DNA test), Factor V R2 (DNA test) or other. Are the results sent back to you directly as a consumer? Or do you purchase additional services such as a physician's interpretation of the results?

What consumers want are genetic tests for metabolism and health. Doctors used genetic testing when patients were concerned about diagnosing inherited diseases. Today, the general consumer of healthcare and healthcare alternative medicine wants genetic testing for general healthcare in the absence of a specific disease. Consumers want to know how to handle the risks they might have inherited to delay or prevent what happened to their grandparents. Also parents of children and couples worried about fertility issues also want these types of tests. Genetic testing shouldn't be used to screen people out of insurance, employment, or anything else.

Health screening should be focused on matching people to the best possible foods, nutraceuticals, and medicines when and if needed. It should be an inclusive not an exclusive process. Like personnel departments that focus on screening out applicants, genetic testing should not be used to screen people out or to exclude based on genetic risks. Instead, it should be used to draw people into learning about taking responsibility for their own health habits such as choosing the right foods. It's all about choice, like the science of nutrition.

Genetic tests were used on people who suffered from rare genetic disease. Consumers are worried about claims by companies that sell DNA tests to the public. Presently, consumers are asking the FDA to review tests before they are sold to the public or to physicians. The FDA reviews drugs and other medical appliances, why not DNA tests or other health screening tests sold to consumers? Should the government be reviewing these tests?

What do you think? Or should the tests be monitored by the companies offering them? Or should the approach be to the tests similar to vitamins and minerals found in health food stores? What side will you take? Do you have enough information to even begin to take sides? Who runs and regulates the DNA testing companies that may or may not be headed by physicians and geneticists?

Testing DNA for ancestry would not have the same impact on someone's health as testing DNA for a specific disease marker. Still, the people doing the testing should have the same qualifications. What about the people doing the interpreting? What stance do you take? Then there's the question of privacy which is essential.

If you're testing for DNA ancestry, you might want to meet your DNA match to correspond with online. If you're testing for a disease marker, you want privacy. You may want to join a support group of families with similar DNA markers for the specific risk or disease you've inherited. You want meetings held in a hospital or some other private, medical setting. Personal issues come up.

Research the various associations of physicians, such as the American Academy of Family Physicians and other similar groups. You can find opinions there. You can bring in lawyers who want to make sure laws are put into effect to keep employers and insurers from using your results to terminate your job or kick you off of health or life insurance plans if your genes put you at risk.

Set up groups made up of advisories of experts that include consumer groups. What consumers with no science background can do is to work with the US Department of Health and Human Services to monitor various panels of experts. Some people want regulations to change. Others don't. There are hundreds of groups out there who advise the US Dept. of Health on what policies they 'should' adopt.

Consumers ask for reviews. Experts ask for reviews. Consumers don't want their vitamins taken away from health food stores. In the midst of it all are the wonderful DNA tests. Talk to pharmacists as well. If you're having adverse reactions to drugs, you eagerly want a DNA test you can take at home as a consumer. What I like about Genelex Corporation's drug metabolism test is that the test can tell you whether your body is taking too long to break down the drugs you're consuming. Consumers need that kind of calmness that comes from knowing personal physicians aren't prescribing too much of what you may or may not need. Maybe you're worrying about your pharmacist giving you the wrong medicine or dosage. Whatever you're concern, a home DNA test is a tool for consumers.

Monitoring your own health is your responsibility, not merely your doctor's. You can get DNA tests sent to your home or scans from clinics. Prescription drugs are available on the Internet. How your body will metabolize what you put into it is important. Are you becoming your own doctor? Is the average consumer becoming more knowledgeable? Or is it more accurate to say most people haven't an inkling of what DNA is?

Pharamcogenetics and nutrigenomics offer tools to consumers. The movement is towards taking charge of your own healthcare. Are doctors worried consumers are taking money away from them? Do tests create more problems than they solve? What happens when scans or other types of tests show non-existent problems?

Research what comes out of the National Institutes of Health. Consumers want to know what the results of their tests mean and how they can apply the information in practical ways. Who interprets the tests? Who is reviewing genetic tests sent directly to consumers and physicians? Right now, it's the consumer's 'job' to ask these questions. If you don't know what vitamins to take, perhaps you need a DNA test to tell you what vitamins work best with your individual genes.

DNA tests seek out mutations in the genes. If a mutation is only remotely associated with a risk, do you ignore it or customize your food and vitamins to the mutation that is only remotely connected to the risk? What action do you take as a consumer? You talk to a physician who knows about genes and your particular risk or you go to a genetics counselor. If you have certain forms of a gene that results in cancer of a certain area of your body by a certain age, you take action right away. Some mutations are associated with disease and some are not, such as certain ancestry markers.

Some genes account for only a tiny percentage of certain cancers. Not everyone needs to be tested. If you have a family reason to be tested, then get tested. If one of your siblings or parents has an inheritable disease, get tested. You can check out Myriad Genetics based in Utah regarding their breast and ovarian cancer tests, available only through doctors. Their Web site is at: http://www.myriad.com/. Or contact them at: Myriad Genetic Laboratories, Inc. | 320 Wakara Way, SLC UT 84108-1214

The Controversy over Whether Genetic Tests should be Sold to the Public

Professionals working in molecular genetics may be divided among those who think genetic tests should be sold to the general consumer and those who think they should not. The professionals who think genetic tests should not be sold to the public may underestimate the intelligence of the public's drive to learn as much as possible about their own genes—the DNA, ancestry, health response to medicine and chemicals in their environment, their response to prescription and over-the-counter drugs, and their response to food, nutraceuticals and other supplements.

Those who are against selling genetic tests to the public fear that genetic testing is way too complex for the average consumer to understand. The average consumer consists of the person who says "it's way over my head," or "my eyes are glazing over" when you mention anything scientific, and the individual who wants to learn as much as possible about his or her own DNA, health, ancestry, and genetic response to food. Most consumers only need to be told that more than a hundred mutations can cause a specific disorder or disease. Average consumers can understand that. Those who underestimate the intelligence and desire to learn of an individual about his or her own health or the health of children and parents usually are the ones who are first to speak out in censorship of a consumer's right to learn all that is possible to learn at the moment about his own genes.

When a consumer is told that negative results don't always signal health, he or she is intelligent to understand that plain English or any language statement. It's a learning process. Some genetics companies are in direct marketing. Some test DNA only for ancestry. Other genetics companies test for genetic responses to drugs or for various genetic health risks that can be helped by changes in diet. The aim of these companies is cooperation. That means cooperation between patient, physician, genetics counselor, dietician or nutritionist and anyone else involved in the healthcare team working with the patient.

In fact in genetics testing, patients are really clients seeking information, feedback, and recommendations for changes in lifestyle and diet. In drug response genetic testing, the client wants to know how his or her body metabolizes the prescription or over-the-counter medicines used. The whole idea of genetic testing is to bring the healthcare team closer to the healthcare consumer. Instead of a one-size-fits all attitude with drugs, foods, or nutraceuticals, or the usual five to fifteen minute consultation with a doctor, the consumer can have the chance to learn everything publicly available about how his or her genes respond to food, drugs, chemicals in the environment, or lifestyle changes.

If a genetics testing company markets cancer tests, it should have the responsibility to let the patient know that the tests are meant for specific people with specific familial cancers and not for the entire consumer population. When a genetics company takes a family history, it opens doors to the individual not only to explore a familial inherited disease or risk, but the entire history and ancestry of the person's family and the DNA of the family members.

Individuals need to learn that there could be more than one gene involved. So teaching consumers about their DNA and genes is important. Classes could be springing up to train people what to expect before they undergo testing. It's a matter of learning and teaching. This is one more way to make use of retired professionals and other scientists and physicians or genetics counselors working in molecular genetics—helping consumers learn what they can expect from testing.

Consumers need to learn about how important it is to sequence certain genes from many family members. Consumers need to get in touch with affected family members and form a support group for DNA testing, perhaps creating a time capsule for future generations with genetic information resulting from testing.

Most consumers go to their family doctors first. Yet how many family physicians are interested in, let alone trained in molecular genetics? Not so many. Most physicians may not interpret a genetic test correctly because they haven't been trained to do so. In may be that the consumer is the first person to request training be set up to show physicians how to interpret genetic tests, especially for such diseases as cancer. Consumers have more power as a group. So consumers need to become involved, work together as an organization, and make sure not only the physicians are trained, but also themselves as consumers of genetic testing. Perhaps the physician and consumer can learn together in groups set up for both, where at a point, physician and consumer meet together. Will this present the physician differently in the eyes of the patient? Not really. The science is new enough so that consumer and patient could learn together to unravel the mysteries of genetics not unlike checking the clues in a mystery novel.

Consumers need to read more medical journals such as the New England Journal of Medicine. Spend some time in the library of your local medical school reading about how physicians interpret genetic testing. Look at surveys. As of now, not too many general consumers from the public at large even know what DNA is. So you have to educate yourself, perhaps as a new hobby. First find out what DNA is. Look it up in the dictionary.

Then start reading magazine articles about genetic testing. Look on the Web at the testing companies. Then you can graduate to reading articles in medical journals. The gap between the physician and the consumer needs to be narrowed at least when it comes to your own DNA and genetic testing for the things consumers put into their body such as food and prescribed or over-the-counter medicines, supplements such as herbs, and other nutraceuticals.

Everyone talks about the consumer's consent to testing. The problem is that the consumer needs to be given information. If you're going to eat 'smarter' you have to become informed first. If you have an inheritable risk or disease, you need to understand everything you can find that is publicly accessible about the risk, the disease, or the genes involved. Material is online, but is it credible? There are always the articles in medical journals, but can you understand the terminology? If not, look up the terms in glossaries and dictionaries. Make a list of terms and learn how to make the journal articles understandable in plain language.

Think about risk for a moment. Your risk could change. How are you going to receive the information from genetic testing? What are you going to do about it as far as changing your lifestyle, diet, or medicines? If you are concerned how your family might react to genetic testing, ask them whether they would change their food choices or other lifestyle changes based on the information. You can always keep the information private, but it could save the lives of family members to get tested and to change what can be changed, such as food choices or exercise routines.

Most consumers worry more about discrimination in employment and health insurance due to companies finding out their genetic risks. Privacy must be kept, and information only given to the consumer of the testing, not his employer or health insurance company. It's nobody's business but your own as far as your genetic information. So, measures to keep out strangers from using your genes against you must be in order. That's why numbers instead of names work better with testing.

The big issue is accuracy. If so many physicians cannot correctly interpret a genetic test and advise their patients, more training is needed for the physicians and the patients. It's a case of whose watching the watchers. Who is going to review the genetic testing itself as to accuracy? What if the tests are not accurate? Right now nobody is reviewing the testing companies other than themselves. Nobody is reporting directly to the consumer after checking the accuracy of the genetic tests. And nobody is reporting directly to the physician with that same information.

If you're going to get tested, at least learn as much as most professional genetic counselors know about interpreting your tests. It can be done without going back to school for a graduate degree in molecular genetics. The information is available to the public from libraries, the Internet, databases, and medical school libraries, journals, and professional articles. Many are on the Web in PDF files. Subscribe to the journals or read them in libraries and learn how to interpret your own tests. Then form a consumer's group to watch the watchers. Learn how to check the accuracy of tests done by the testing companies.

You have to become involved in your own healthcare and nutrition. Take charge and take responsibility. Consumers can't be passive. You won't know how your body responds to food or medicine or lifestyle changes until symptoms appear. Start by looking at the health of your family members and realizing what is inheritable, and what you can do to help yourself if you've inherited what they have or will get.

The first step for consumers is to start learning about DNA and genetic testing just as they have learned about genealogy and family history. Classes online or in adult education can be set up as well as support groups and organizations of consumers. The second step is to form a group to review the accuracy of information that comes with your genetic tests. Invite physicians and other healthcare professionals to join with consumers and become a team. Don't let separation between those with scientific knowledge and those without become a barrier to reviewing accuracy of information. When several physicians or geneticists band together to review the accuracy of information provided with genetic testing, what might happen is that the group then becomes made up only of professionals. When consumers group together, they can include professionals, but would never ban someone from the group because of professional training in the field they are watching.

So consumers need to create a group to review the accuracy of information that comes with genetic tests. And that same group needs to make sure education exists for consumers. You need to set up classes to train consumers in how to understand the results of their genetic testing and how to review the accuracy of the information given along with the genetic tests. If trained physicians can't correctly interpret a genetic test for their patients in certain cases, it's time for consumers to take charge of their own healthcare education. Okay, you can't do surgery on yourself, but you can learn to read the information provided with genetic tests. And having read the information, you can learn also to question the accuracy of that information. Consumers can read not only the medical journal articles usually found in medical school and university libraries open to the public, publications such as the ***New England Journal of Medicine***, but also some of the more popular articles in magazines that go to physicians such as ***Physician's Weekly***.

All this autodidact education can be achieved with consumers involvement and support groups if people are interested enough to involve a wide range of members or participants. Genetic training should be available to everyone equally and widely available through the internet, through senior centers, classrooms focused on adult education, through hospitals and HMO programs, and through the genetic testing companies.

In the magazine, *Physician's Weekly*, October 7, 2002, Vol. XIX, No. 38, the article in Point/Counterpoint, titled, *"Should genetic tests be sold directly to the public?"* featured Howard Coleman, CEO, Genelex Corp., Redmond, Washington and Kimberly A. Quaid, PhD, Professor of Clinical, Medical, and Molecular Genetics, Clinical Psychiatry, and Clinical Medicine, Indiana University School of Medicine. Coleman's response was yes, and Quaid's response was no. See the article, copyrighted 2002 by *Physician's Weekly*, reprinted below with permission.

Should genetic tests be sold directly to the public?

Howard Coleman, CEO, Genelex Corp., Redmond, Washington.

YES Every person has the right to know his or her genetic information, and the right not to share it. People have legitimate privacy concerns about their genetic information being loose in the medical records system, fearing for their jobs or insurance if it gets into the wrong hands. Physicians are also concerned, and don't want to risk compromising a patient's privacy. This contributes to their reluctance to order genetic tests.

There are compelling reasons for people to obtain reliable genetic information, whether they go through their doctors or not. According to a 1998 JAMA article, more than 100,000 deaths occur annually due to adverse drug reactions, along with an additional 2.2 million serious events that require hospital stays. These are not medical mishaps, as they occur within the labeled use of drugs.

When physicians begin to learn the genotype of their patients they will begin to solve this problem. The practice of their clinical art will be improved because in many instances the genotype of their patient trumps the many other characteristics they do know.

Despite the facts that science has known for the past half century that people react differently to drugs, doctors have been unable to put genetic testing into practice for the benefit of their patients. Doctors lack sufficient training in pharmacogenetics and drug metabolism. For example, most doctors don't know that genotyping for Coumadin metabolism is available, and that it will help patients avoid adverse reactions with this drug.

Adverse drug reactions kill many people in the U.S., but the threat goes largely unrecognized. Making gene tests available directly to patients not only provides a valuable service, but helps push the medical community into the 21st century era of personalized and evidence-based medicine.

Kimberly A. Quaid, PhD, Professor of Clinical, Medical, and Molecular Genetics, Clinical Psychiatry, and Clinical Medicine Indiana University School of Medicine

NO No. Genetic testing is far too complex for lay people to tackle on their own. For example, more than 100 mutations can cause cystic fibrosis, and most genetic tests only cover a small subset of these. But most lay people don't understand that negative results are not necessarily a clean bill of health.

The announcement last spring that Myriad Genetics would direct market cancer tests was particularly troubling, because such tests are only appropriate for a small number of individuals with certain familial cancers. The complex protocol includes taking a detailed family history, then finding and sequencing the gene from affected relatives (and there may be more than one gene).

Individuals who hear about such tests might approach their family physicians, but research shows that many are not trained in genetics. A paper in the NEJM, which looked at physicians ordering a test for a particular cancer, found that one third of these physicians interpreted the test incorrectly. One can assume that if physicians have trouble interpreting the results, patients will fare far worse. One survey found that fewer than 26% of Americans know what DNA is.

Geneticists believe testing should be preceded by informed consent. For consent to be informed, the patient must understand the disorder for which they are being tested, their current risk, how their risk might change as a result of testing, the ramifications of their being tested for their families and spouses, and the possibility of discrimination should third parties get their hands on this information.

Finally, no mechanism exists to review the accuracy of information provided with genetic tests to either health-care professionals or consumers. Individuals who get tested without professional counseling may buy trouble with their test results.

In our recent email interview of August 19, 2003, Howard Coleman added, ""I agree with Dr. Quaid when the testing concerns the grave medical conditions caused by genetic disease and we don't offer those tests to the general public. The testing we do provide can help both the physician and the individual understand their ability to metabolize drugs which can help to prevent adverse drug reactions and how to optimize their diet."

Scientists and Physicians Comment on Pharmacogenetics

Why would the average consumer of health care want to have drug reaction testing, known as pharmacogenetic testing? The field is new, and still emerging. According to (reprinted with permission) Genelex's "Health and DNA" Web site (copyright 2003) at: http://www.healthanddna.com/, "The relatively new and emerging fields of pharmacogenetics studies how differences in individual genetic makeup affect the processing of drugs. We have known for about a half-century that individuals respond to the same drug and dosage in very different ways because of genetic variations called polymorphisms. Research shows that of all the clinical factors such as age, sex, weight, general health and liver function that alter a patient's response to drugs, genetic factors are the most important. Genelex is the first firm in the world to offer genetic drug reaction testing directly to the public." What I like about Genelex is that they also offer DNA testing for nutritional genetics, drug reaction testing, ancestry DNA testing, and DNA identity testing.

DNA traditionally had been used to identify people, mostly in forensic or paternity or relationship cases. Then a few years ago, companies began to test DNA for ancestry, which appeals also to genealogists, family historians, and oral historians.

The use of DNA outside of court rooms and forensic laboratories and outside of government and university databases brought DNA to consumers of health care as well as to genealogists interested in molecular genealogy. University laboratories and archaeology research institutes began using the science of archaeogenetics.

Anthropologists who looked at HLA markers, those leukocytes or white blood cells and physicians or scientists who were interested in tissue typing for blood, marrow, and organ transplant donors worked with DNA to identify similar matches, people whose tissues and blood or marrow typing matched close enough for a transplant to take.

You had scientists who studied ancient DNA from fossils and mummies expand the science of archaeogenetics and population geneticists studying migrations of ancient peoples and the routes they took. When ancient and present day comparisons of genetic markers left trails that matched with archaeological relics, new branches of molecular genetics grew.

The science is still emerging, using DNA testing in more ways. Now, we have nutrition and genetics and drug testing and genetics. And there's so much more to arrive that will be available to the general consumer of healthcare, ancestry searching, and identity. From being a spectator in life watching new avenues of DNA testing unfold, the consumer now has the chance to become more involved in participating in and learning about how many ways DNA testing can benefit an individual at any age.

When I went back to Genelex's Web site to explore more material on DNA testing for a variety of purposes, I realized, the consumer has more choices than ever before and still more on the horizon. DNA testing is all about nourishment. From nutrigenomics to drug reaction testing, strategies for better health is being covered from all angles.

Perhaps you—as a consumer—want a healthier eating guideline customized to your genetic signature. Maybe you'd like a report on how your genes (and body) respond to certain chemicals, medicines, or substances. Whether it's a prescription drug or specific medicines or supplements that you buy over the counter, several genes are tested to see how your body metabolizes the substance.

Not every gene in your body is tested to see how they respond to food or medicine—just specific genes and markers. The science is new and changing, but the future is attractive to general consumers. You don't need a science background to begin your research on how your own body responds to what you put into it and what comes it from the environment. To begin, consumers need to become more involved in learning about what scientists and physicians are researching and why, and how all these new findings apply to you.

To become more involved as a consumer means being able to access information that evaluates the research, that finds credibility or flaws, and that helps you take more responsibility in your own maintenance. That's why DNA testing may open doors. Even with guarded caution, the benefits are to be explored and discussed. If you have already had your DNA tested for ancestry or identity, consider these new ways in which DNA testing can help you draw up a plan for eating and for any way you take care of your body—from exercise planning and nutrition to medicines and supplements if and when you need them, to making lifestyle changes for better health.

Consumers can learn a lot from news releases, including learning to understand where to begin to educate themselves about their genes. Some of these releases come from universities engaged in research, some from laboratories and genetic testing companies, some from the government, and from other scientific sources. Professionals in molecular genetics and in healthcare need to understand that an open door policy for public education, teaching oneself about DNA is good. To become more informed leads to becoming more involved in consumer's groups for understanding what "gene hunters" are doing.

Science has become so technical that most scientific journal articles are not understood by most consumers without science training. There has to be a mid-way point. So far, it's the media that translates scientific terminology into plain language for the consumer. Going one step farther, the medical journalist translates the scientific journals into articles and books whereby people with no science background can learn about their genes.

Finally, learning about how one's genes respond to food or drugs is another rung up on the ladder of self-education about how your body works. That's why there's the mass media for the consumer, the popular medical magazines that bring the consumer closer to healthcare professionals, and finally, the scientific and medical journal articles discussing the research. At the top are the evaluators who let the consumers know which research studies were flawed, and that usually filters down through the mass media.

What some scientists call 'snake oil' may either be harmful or may be a forgotten remedy based on plants that worked. For example, honey, cinnamon, and sesame oil. All three will resist bacteria and in the ancient past were used on minor wounds. A century ago colloidal silver was used on scratches to keep out bacteria.

In the Civil War days, it was used on wounds. Today, you can still make your own, inexpensively, but be careful buying brands containing aluminum. In the dentist's chair, colloidal silver mouthwash works as well as some of the more recent remedies such as washing your mouth with harsh substances that can cause ulcers in the mouth. The point is to check out the mechanisms that review accuracy in whatever you read. If you go the homeopathic or naturopathic route, make sure what you use does no harm for your individual genetic response. How do you metabolize what goes into your body? Genetic testing can help here.

When it comes to genetic testing, you can learn a lot from news releases—at least as a starting point in your research and education about your genes. Bioscience communicators have a role to play as interpreters between consumer and scientist. When I took my master's degree in English with a writing emphasis, it was through a graduate scholarship award in science writing. In genetics, being the communicator means bridging the gap between the growing body of knowledge in science and the consumer who might not even know what DNA is. If you have no science knowledge, start by reading press releases to open the first set of doors to understanding more about your genes, markers, and DNA.

8

How To Interview People If You Are Ghostwriting Memoirs, Life Stories, Unique Experiences, Social History, Or Current Issues

Step 1

When you interview, ask for facts and concrete details. Look for statistics, and research whether statistics are deceptive in your case.

Step 2

To write a plan, write one sentence for each topic that moves the story or piece forward. Then summarize for each topic in a paragraph. Use dialogue at least in every third paragraph.

Step 3

Look for the following facts or headings to organize your plan for a biography or life story.

1. PROVERB. Ask the people you interview what would be their proverb or slogan if they had to create/invent a slogan that fit themselves or their aspirations: One slogan might be something like the seventies ad for cigarettes, "We've come a long way, baby," to signify ambition. Only look for an original slogan.

2. PURPOSE. Ask the people you interview or a biography, for what purpose is or was their journey? Is or was it equality in the workplace or something per-

sonal and different such as dealing with change—downsizing, working after retirement, or anything else?

3.   IMPRINT. Ask what makes an imprint or impact on people's lives and what impact the people you're interviewing want to make on others?

4.   STATISTICS: How deceptive are they? How can you use them to focus on reality?

5.   How have the people that you're interviewing influenced changes in the way people or corporations function?

6.   To what is the person aspiring?

7.   What kind of communication skills does the person have and how are these skills received? Are the communication skills male or female, thinking or feeling, yin or yang, soft or steeled, and are people around these people negative or positive about those communication skills?

8.   What new styles is the person using? What kind of motivational methods, structure, or leadership? Is the person a follower or leader? How does the person match his or her personality to the character of a corporation or interest?

9.   How does the person handle change?

10. How is the person reinforced?

Once you have titles and summarized paragraphs for each segment of your story, you can more easily flesh out the story by adding dialogue and description to your factual information. Look for differences in style between the people you interview? How does the person want to be remembered?

Is the person a risk taker or cautious for survival? Does the person identify with her job or the people involved in the process of doing the work most creatively or originally?

Does creative expression take precedence over processes of getting work out to the right place at the right time? Does the person want his ashes to spell the words "re-invent yourself" where the sea meets the shore? This is a popular concept appearing in various media.

Search the Records in the Family History Library of Salt Lake City, Utah

Make use of the database online at the Family History Library of Salt Lake City, Utah. Or visit the branches in many locations. The Family History Library (FHL) is known worldwide as the focal point of family history records preservation.

The FHL collection contains more than 2.2 million rolls of microfilmed genealogical records, 742,000 microfiche, 300,000 books, and 4,500 periodicals that represent data collected from over 105 countries. You don't have to be a member of any particular church or faith to use the library or to go online and search the records.

Family history records owe a lot to the invention of writing. And then there is oral history, but someone needs to transcribe oral history to record and archive them for the future.

Interestingly, isn't it a coincidence that writing is 6,000 years old and DNA that existed 6,000 years ago first reached such crowded conditions in the very cities that had first used writing extensively to measure accounting and trade had very little recourse but to move on to new areas where there were far less people and less use of writing?

A lot of major turning points occurred 6,000 years ago—the switch to a grain-based diet from a meat and root diet, the use of bread and fermented grain beverages, making of oil from plants, and the rise of religions based on building "god houses" in the centers of town in areas known as the "cereal belt" around the world.

Six thousand years ago in India we have the start of the Sanskrit writings, the cultivation of grain. In China, we have the recording of acupuncture points for medicine built on energy meridians that also show up in the blue tattoos of the Ice Man fossil "Otsi" in the Alps—along the same meridians as the Chinese acupuncture points.

At 6,000 years ago the Indo European languages spread out across Europe. Mass migrations expanded by the Danube leaving pottery along the trade routes that correspond to the clines and gradients of gene frequency coming out of the cereal belts.

Then something happened. There was an agricultural frontier cutting off the agriculturists from the hunters. Isn't it a coincidence that the agricultural frontiers or barriers also are genetic barriers at least to some degree?

Oral History

Here's how to systematically collect, record, and preserve living peoples' testimonies about their own experiences. After you record in audio and/or video the highlights of anyone's experiences, try to verify your findings. See whether you can check any facts in order to find out whether the person being recorded is making up the story or whether it really did happen.

This is going to be difficult unless you have witnesses or other historical records. Once you have verified your findings to the best of your ability, note whether the findings have been verified. Then analyze what you found. Put the oral history recordings in an accurate historical context.

Mark the recordings with the dates and places. Watch where you store your findings so scholars in the future will be able to access the transcript or recording and convert the recording to another, newer technology. For instance, if you have a transcript on paper, have it saved digitally on a disk and somewhere else on tape and perhaps a written transcript on acid-free good paper in case technology moves ahead before the transcript or recording is converted to the new technology.

For example, if you only put your recording on a phonograph record, within a generation or two, there may not be any phonographs around to play the record. The same goes for CDs, DVDs and audio or video tapes.

So make sure you have a readable paper copy to be transcribed or scanned into the new technology as well as the recordings on disk and tape. For example, if you record someone's experiences in a live interview with your video camera, use a cable to save the video in the hard disk of a computer and then burn the file to a CD or DVD.

Keep a copy of audio tape and a copy of regular video tape—all in a safe place such as a time capsule, and make a copy for various archives in libraries and university oral history preservation centers. Be sure scholars in the future can find a way to enjoy the experiences in your time capsule, scrapbook, or other storage device for oral histories.

Use your DNA testing results to add more information to a historical record. As an interviewer with a video camera and/or audio tape recorder, your task is to record as a historical record what the person who you are interviewing recollects.

The events move from the person being interviewed to you, the interviewer, and then into various historical records. In this way you can combine results of DNA testing with actual memories of events. If it's possible, also take notes or have someone take notes in case the tape doesn't pick up sounds clearly.

I had the experience of having a video camera battery go out in spite of all precautions when I was interviewing someone, and only the audio worked. So keep a backup battery on hand whether you use a tape recorder or a video camera. If at all possible, have a partner bring a spare camera and newly recharged battery. A fully charged battery left overnight has a good chance of going out when you need it.

Writing Skits from Oral and Personal History Transcripts

Emphasize the commitment to family and faith. To create readers' and media attention to an oral history, it should have some redemptive value to a universal audience. That's the most important point. Make your oral history simple and earthy. Write about real people who have values, morals, and a faith in something greater than themselves that is equally valuable to readers or viewers.

Publishers who buy an oral history written as a book on its buzz value are buying simplicity. It is simplicity that sells and nothing else but simplicity. This is true for oral histories, instructional materials, and fiction. It's good storytelling to say it simply.

Simplicity means the oral history or memoirs book or story gives you all the answers you were looking for in your life in exotic places, but found it close by. What's the great proverb that your oral history is telling the world?

Is it to stand on your own two feet and put bread on your own table for your family? That's the moral point, to pull your own weight, and pulling your own weight is a buzz word that sells oral histories and fiction that won't preach, but instead teach and reach through simplicity.

That's the backbone of the oral historian's new media. Buzz means the story is simple to understand. You make the complex easier to grasp. And buzz means you can sell your story or book, script or narrative by focusing on the values of simplicity, morals, faith, and universal values that hold true for everyone.

Doing the best to take care of your family sells and is buzz appeal, hot stuff in the publishing market of today and in the oral history archives. This is true, regardless of genre. Publishers go through fads every two years—angel books, managing techniques books, computer home-based business books, novels about ancient historical characters or tribes, science fiction, children's programming, biography, and oral history transcribed into a book or play.

The genres shift emphasis, but values are consistent in the bestselling books. Perhaps your oral history will be simple enough to become a bestselling book or script. In the new media, simplicity is buzz along with values.

Oral history, like best-selling novels and true stories is built on simplicity, values, morals, and commitment. Include how one person dealt with about trends. Focus your own oral history about life in the lane of your choice. Develop one central issue and divide that issue into a few important questions that highlight or focus on that one central issue.

When you write or speak a personal history either alone or in an interview, you focus on determining the order of your life story. Don't use flashbacks. Focus on the highlights and turning points. Organize what you'll say or write. An autobiography deals in people's relationships. Your autobiography deals as much with what doesn't change—the essentials—as what life changes you and those around you go through.

Your personal history should be more concrete than abstract. You want the majority of people to understand what you mean. Say what you mean, and mean what you say. More people understand concrete details than understand abstract ideas.

How to Gather Personal or Medical Histories
Use the following sequence when gathering oral/aural histories:

1.   Develop one central issue and divide that issue into a few important questions that highlight or focus on that one central issue.

2.   Write out a plan just like a business plan for your oral history project. You may have to use that plan later to ask for a grant for funding, if required. Make a list of all your products that will result from the oral history when it's done.

3.   Write out a plan for publicity or public relations and media relations. How are you going to get the message to the public or special audiences?

4.   Develop a budget. This is important if you want a grant or to see how much you'll have to spend on creating an oral history project.

5.   List the cost of video taping and editing, packaging, publicity, and help with audio or special effects and stock shot photos of required.

6.   What kind of equipment will you need? List that and the time slots you give to each part of the project. How much time is available? What are your deadlines?

7. What's your plan for a research? How are you going to approach the people to get the interviews? What questions will you ask?

8. Do the interviews. Arrive prepared with a list of questions. It's okay to ask the people the kind of questions they would like to be asked. Know what dates the interviews will cover in terms of time. Are you covering the economic depression of the thirties? World Wars? Fifties? Sixties? Pick the time parameters.

9. Edit the interviews so you get the highlights of experiences and events, the important parts. Make sure what's important to you also is important to the person you interviewed.

10. Find out what the interviewee wants to emphasize perhaps to highlight events in a life story. Create a video-biography of the highlights of one person's life or an oral history of an event or series of events.

11. Process audio as well as video, and make sure you have written transcripts of anything on audio and/or video in case the technology changes or the tapes go bad.

12. Save the tapes to compact disks, DVDs, a computer hard disk and several other ways to preserve your oral history time capsule. Donate any tapes or CDs to appropriate archives, museums, relatives of the interviewee, and one or more oral history libraries. They are usually found at universities that have an oral history department and library such as UC Berkeley and others.

13. Check the Web for oral history libraries at universities in various states and abroad.

14. Evaluate what you have edited. Make sure the central issue and central questions have been covered in the interview. Find out whether newspapers or magazines want summarized transcripts of the audio and/or video with photos.

15. Contact libraries, archives, university oral history departments and relevant associations and various ethnic genealogy societies that focus on the subject matter of your central topic.

16. Keep organizing what you have until you have long and short versions of your oral history for various archives and publications. Contact magazines and newspapers to see whether editors would assign reporters to do a story on the oral history project.

17. Create a scrapbook with photos and summarized oral histories. Write a synopsis of each oral history on a central topic or issue. Have speakers give public presentations of what you have for each person interviewed and/or for the entire project using highlights of several interviews with the media for publicity. Be sure your project is archived properly and stored in a place devoted to oral history archives and available to researchers and authors.

Oral History Techniques

1. Begin with easy to answer questions that don't require you explore and probe deeply in your first question. Focus on one central issue when asking questions. Don't use abstract questions. A plain question would be "What's your purpose?" An abstract question with connotations would be "What's your crusade?" Use questions with denotations instead of connotations. Keep questions short and plain—easy to understand. Examples would be, "What did you want to accomplish? How did you solve those problems? How did you find closure?" Ask the familiar "what, when, who, where, how, and why."

2. First research written or visual resources before you begin to seek an oral history of a central issue, experience, or event.

3. Who is your intended audience?

4. What kind of population niche or sample will you target?

5. What means will you select to choose who you will interview? What group of people will be central to your interview?

6. Write down how you'll explain your project. Have a script ready so you don't digress or forget what to say on your feet.

7. Consult oral history professionals if you need more information. Make sure what you write in your script will be clear to understand by your intended audience.

8. Have all the equipment you need ready and keep a list of what you'll use and the cost. Work up your budget.

9. Choose what kind of recording device is best—video, audio, multimedia, photos, and text transcript. Make sure your video is broadcast quality. I use a Sony Digital eight (high eight) camera.

10. Make sure from cable TV stations or news stations that what type of video and audio you choose ahead of time is broadcast quality.

11. Make sure you have an external microphone and also a second microphone as a second person also tapes the interview in case the quality of your camera breaks down. You can also keep a tape recorder going to capture the audio in case your battery dies.

12. Make sure your battery is fully charged right before the interview. Many batteries die down after a day or two of nonuse.

13. Test all equipment before the interview and before you leave your office or home. I've had batteries go down unexpectedly and happy there was another person ready with another video camera waiting and also an audio tape version going.

14. Make sure the equipment works if it's raining, hot, cold, or other weather variations. Test it before the interview. Practice interviewing someone on your equipment several times to get the hang of it before you show up at the interview.

15. Make up your mind how long the interview will go before a break and use tape of that length, so you have one tape for each segment of the interview. Make several copies of your interview questions.

16. Be sure the interviewee has a copy of the questions long before the interview so the person can practice answering the questions and think of what to say or even take notes. Keep checking your list of what you need to do.

17. Let the interviewee make up his own questions if he wants. Perhaps your questions miss the point. Present your questions first. Then let him embellish the questions or change them as he wants to fit the central issue with his own experiences.

18. Call the person two days and then one day before the interview to make sure the individual will be there on time and understands how to travel to the location. Or if you are going to the person's home, make sure you understand how to get there.

19. Allow yourself one extra hour in case of traffic jams.

20. Choose a quiet place. Turn off cell phones and any ringing noises. Make sure you are away from barking dogs, street noise, and other distractions.

21. Before you interview make sure the person knows he or she is going to be video and audio-taped.

22. If you don't want anyone swearing, make that clear it's for public archives and perhaps broadcast to families.

23. Your interview questions should follow the journalist's information-seeking format of asking, who, what, where, where, how, and why. Oral history is a branch of journalistic research.

24. Let the person talk and don't interrupt. You be the listener and think of oral history as aural history from your perspective.

25. Make sure only one person speaks without being interrupted before someone else takes his turn to speak.

26. Understand silent pauses are for thinking of what to say.

27. Ask one question and let the person gather his thoughts.

28. Finish all your research on one question before jumping to the next question. Keep it organized by not jumping back to the first question after the second is done. Stay in a linear format.

29. Follow up what you can about any one question, finish with it, and move on to the next question without circling back. Focus on listening instead of asking rapid fire questions as they would confuse the speaker.

30. Ask questions that allow the speaker to begin to give a story, anecdote, life experience, or opinion along with facts. Don't ask questions that can be

answered only be yes or no. This is not a courtroom. Let the speaker elaborate with facts and feelings or thoughts.

31. Late in the interview, start to ask questions that explore and probe for deeper answers.

32. Wrap up with how the person solved the problem, achieved results, reached a conclusion, or developed an attitude, or found the answer. Keep the wrap-up on a light, uplifting note.

33. Don't leave the individual hanging in emotion after any intensity of. Respect the feelings and opinions of the person. He or she may see the situation from a different point of view than someone else. So respect the person's right to feel as he does. Respect his need to recollect his own experiences.

34. Interview for only one hour at a time. If you have only one chance, interview for an hour. Take a few minutes break. Then interview for the second hour. Don't interview more than two hours at any one meeting.

35. Use prompts such as paintings, photos, music, video, diaries, vintage clothing, crafts, antiques, or memorabilia when appropriate. Carry the photos in labeled files or envelopes to show at appropriate times in order to prime the memory of the interviewee. For example, you may show a childhood photo and ask "What was it like in that orphanage where these pictures were taken?" Or travel photos might suggest a trip to America as a child, or whatever the photo suggests. For example, "Do you remember when this ice cream parlor inside the ABC movie house stood at the corner of X and Y Street? Did you go there as a teenager? What was your funniest memory of this movie theater or the ice cream store inside back in the fifties?"

36. As soon as the interview is over, label all the tapes and put the numbers in order.

37. A signed release form is required before you can broadcast anything. So have the interviewee sign a release form before the interview.

38. Make sure the interviewee gets a copy of the tape and a transcript of what he or she said on tape. If the person insists on making corrections, send the paper transcript of the tape for correction to the interviewee. Edit the tape as best you can or have it edited professionally.

39. Make sure you comply with all the corrections the interviewee wants changed. He or she may have given inaccurate facts that need to be corrected on the paper transcript.

40. Have the tape edited with the corrections, even if you have to make a tape at the end of the interviewee putting in the corrections that couldn't be edited out or changed.

41. As a last resort, have the interviewee redo the part of the tape that needs correction and have it edited in the tape at the correct place marked on the tape. Keep the paper transcript accurate and up to date, signed with a release form by the interviewee.

42. Oral historians write a journal of field notes about each interview. Make sure these get saved and archived so they can be read with the transcript.

43. Have the field notes go into a computer where someone can read them along with the transcript of the oral history tape or CD.

44. Thank the interviewee in writing for taking the time to do an interview for broadcast and transcript.

45. Put a label on everything you do from the interview to the field notes. Make a file and sub file folders and have everything stored in a computer, in archived storage, and in paper transcript.

46. Make copies and digital copies of all photos and put into the records in a computer. Return originals to owners.

47. Make sure you keep your fingerprints off the photos by wearing white cotton gloves. Use cardboard when sending the photos back and pack securely. Also photocopy the photos and scan the photos into your computer. Treat photos as antique art history in preservation.

48. Make copies for yourself of all photos, tapes, and transcripts. Use your duplicates, and store the original as the master tape in a place that won't be used often, such as a time capsule or safe, or return to a library or museum where the original belongs.

49. Return all original photos to the owners. An oral history archive library or museum also is suitable for original tapes. Use copies only to work from, copy, or distribute.

50. Index your tapes and transcripts. To use oral history library and museum terminology, recordings and transcripts are given "accession numbers."

51. Phone a librarian in an oral history library of a university for directions on how to assign accession numbers to your tapes and transcripts if the materials are going to be stored at that particular library. Store copies in separate places in case of loss or damage.

52. If you don't know where the materials will be stored, use generic accession numbers to label your tapes and transcripts. Always keep copies available for yourself in case you have to duplicate the tapes to send to an institution, museum, or library, or to a broadcast company.

53. Make synopses available to public broadcasting radio and TV stations.

54. Check your facts.

55. Are you missing anything you want to include?

56. Is there some place you want to send these tapes and transcripts such as an ethnic museum, radio show, or TV satellite station specializing in the topics on the tapes, such as public TV stations? Would it be suitable for a world music station? A documentary station?

57. If you need more interviews, arrange them if possible.

58. Give the interviewee a copy of the finished product with the corrections. Make sure the interviewee signs a release form that he or she is satisfied with the corrections and is releasing the tape to you and your project.

59. Store the tapes and transcripts in a library or museum or at a university or other public place where it will be maintained and preserved for many generations and restored when necessary.

60. You can also send copies to a film repository or film library that takes video tapes, an archive for radio or audio tapes for radio broadcast or cable TV.

61. Copies may be sent to various archives for storage that lasts for many generations. Always ask whether there are facilities for restoring the tape. A museum would most likely have these provisions as would a large library that has an oral history library project or section.

62. Make sure the master copy is well protected and set up for long-term storage in a place where it will be protected and preserved.

63. If the oral history is about events in history, various network news TV stations might be interested. Film stock companies may be interested in copies of old photos.

64. Find out from the subject matter what type of archives, repository, or storage museums and libraries would be interested in receiving copies of the oral history tapes and transcripts.

9

Document Recovery for Personal History Time Capsules & Memorabilia

How do you rescue and recover memories from mold using conservation techniques? You transport horizontally and store vertically. Store documents and photos in plastic holders, between sheets of waxed paper, or interleave with acid-free paper. Books are stored spine down. Archive DVDs and CDs in plastic holders and store in plastic crates. To conserve time capsules, according to the American Institute for Conservation of Historic and Artistic Works (AIC), in Washington, DC, neutralize that acid-wracked paper.

Diaries, Bibles, and Old Family Cookbooks

Here's how to "mend conditions" and restore diaries. First make a book jacket for a diary. Put a title and label on the dust jacket with the name of the diary's author and any dates, city, state, or country.

Use acid-free paper for the jacket. Diaries and book jackets are works of art. If torn, mend the diary. Apply a protective plastic wrapper to your valuable dust jacket or give diaries dust jackets in good condition.

Be cautious using bleach, because chlorine fumes will fade the ink and soak through the opposite page to fade that writing. After testing the bleach, if the diary is dingy and dirty, bleach it white on the edges only using diluted bleach that won't fade old ink. Test the bleach first on similar surfaces, such as a blank page in the book.

Repair old diaries, and turn them into heirlooms for families and valuable collectibles. The current price for repairing handwritten diaries and books is about $50 and up per book or bound diary. Better yet, publish diaries as print-on-demand PDF files and print them out as paperback books with covers for families.

Some diaries served as handwritten cookbooks containing recipes created by a particular family cook. For more repair tips on bound diaries-as-cook-books, I recommend the book titled, *How to Wrap a Book*, Fannie Merit Farmer, Boston Cooking School.

How do you repair an old diary or family recipe book to make it more valuable to heirs? You'll often find a bound diary that's torn in the seams. According to Barbara Gelink, of the 1990s Collector's Old Cookbooks Club, San Diego, to repair a book, you take a bottle of Book Saver Glue (or any other book-repairing or wood glue), and spread the glue along the binder.

Run the glue along the seam and edges. Use wax paper to keep the glue from getting where it shouldn't. Put a heavy glass bottle on the inside page to hold it down while the glue dries.

Use either the *finest* grade sand paper or nail polish remover to unglue tape, tags, or stains from a *glossy* cover. Sit away from heat, light, and sparks. Carefully dampen a terry cloth with nail polish remover, lighter, or cleaning fluid and circle gently until the tag and stain are gone. On a *plastic* book cover, use the finest grade of sandpaper.

Memorabilia such as diaries, genealogy materials, books, photos, ivory, sports trophies, cards, discarded library and school books, or fabrics that end up at estate sales or thrift shops may have adhesive price tags.

To bleach the "discarded book stamp" that libraries and schools often use, or any other rubber stamp mark, price, date, or seals on the pages or edges, use regular bleach, like Clorox. It turns the rubber stamp mark white. The household bleach also turns the edges and pages of the book white as new.

To preserve a valuable, tattered dust jacket with tears along the edges, provide extra firmness. Put a protective plastic wrapper on top of the book jacket cover of a diary, especially if it's handwritten.

To collect diaries or family photos, look in garage sales, flea markets, and antique shops. Attend auctions and book fairs. Two recommended auction houses for rare cookbooks include Pacific Book Auction Galleries, 139 Townsend, #305, San Francisco, CA 94107, or Sotheby's, New York, 1334 York Ave., New York, NY 10021. Pacific Book Auction Galleries sometimes puts cookbook collections up for an auction.

Look for old high-school graduation class year books to collect from various high schools or middle schools found in garage and estate sales. Restore them and find out whether there's an alumni association whose members want that book stored where all can access it, such as in a public or school library offering interstate library loans.

Can the diary, recipe book, or school yearbook be restored and digitized on DVDs with permission from those who copyrighted it? If you're into keepsake album making with family history photos, diaries, or recipes, look for cookbooks printed by high school parent-teacher associations. Some old ones may be valuable, but even the one put out by the depression era San Diego High School Parent Teacher Association for the class of 1933-34 is only worth $10.

You can start a family history business specializing in restoring diaries, domestic history journals, school yearbooks, and certain types of personal, rare, or cook books. For example, *Cornucopia*, run by Carol A. Greenberg, has old and rare books emphasizing cooking, food literature, domestic history, household management, herbs, kitchen gardens, hotels, restaurants, etiquette, manners, pastimes, amusements, and needlework.

They search for out-of-print books, and are interested in material from the 19th century through 1940. Write to: Little Treasures at PO Box 742, Woodbury, NY 11797. Greenberg is always grateful for quotations on old, rare, and unusual materials in fine condition.

You could start a collector's old diaries and photos club. Marge Rice is a pioneer genealogist who created a hobby of returning heirloom photos to their families of origin. See the related article at: http://www.ancestry.com/library/view/ancmag/7643.asp. Or digitize photos for the Web. See the instructional site on digitizing photos for the Web at: http://www.firstmonday.dk/issues/issue8_1/garner/.

Some bound handwritten diaries were purchased as blank or lined notebooks. People who collect autographs may also be interested in diaries of authors. For example, the published diary novel titled *One Day Some Schlemiel Will Marry Me* is a diary that ended up as a published first person life story novel. Other diaries end up as cookbooks.

Are diaries worth as much as rare cookbooks? How much are the thousands of rare cookbooks worth today? A helpful guide is the Price Guide to Cookbooks & Recipe Leaflets, 1990, by Linda J. Dickinson, published by Collector Books, at PO Box 3009, Paducah, KY 42002-3009.

See Bibliography of American Cookery Books, 1742-1860. It's based on Waldo Lincoln's American Cookery Books 1742-1860, by Eleanor Lowenstein. Over 800 books and pamphlets are listed. Order from Oak Knoll Books & Press, 414 Delaware St., Newcastle, Delaware 19720.

Louis & Clark Booksellers specialize in rare and out-of-print cookery, gastronomy, wine and beverages, baking, restaurants, domestic history, etiquette, and travel books. They're at 2402 Van Hise Avenue, Madison, WI 53705. Cook books are much more in demand than diaries, unless the author has celebrity status.

Make copies of diaries. Work with the photocopies when you decipher the writing. Store your old diaries in a dry, cool place. Lining the storage place with plastic that's sealed will keep out vermin, moisture, and bugs. Without moisture, you can keep out the mildew and mold. Store duplicates away from originals.

Was something placed in a diary on a certain page, such as a dried rose, letter, farmer's wheat stain, or a special book mark? What meaning did it have? Look for clues for a time frame. Date the diary. List the date it was begun and when it was ended if you can. List the geographic location of the events in the diary and the writer's travels.

Of what kind of materials is the diary made? Is it improvised, created at low cost by the author? Or is it fancy and belonging to someone of wealth? What is the layout like? Does it show the education of the writer or anything personal? Was it a farmer's almanac, captain's log or sailor's calendar, personal journal or if recent, a Web log (blog)?

What was the writing tool, a quill or a pencil? What's the handwriting like? What century or years? Is it full of details, maps, corsages, and pictures? What is its central message? Do you see patterns or mainly listed facts?

Transcribe the diary with your computer. Read it into a camcorder or on audio tape. It's now oral history. What historical events influenced the writing of the diary? What's the social history? What language is it in or dialect? Are there vital records such as wills or deeds to real estate mentioned in the diary? You've now mended, restored, and conserved a life story and a pattern on the quilt of humanity.

Acid Paper:

Here's how to prevent acidic paper damage in your paper memorabilia or on your items stored against paper. According to author, Betty Walsh, Conservator, BC Archives, Canada and the Walsh's information and Web site at: http://palimpsest.stanford.edu/waac/wn/wn10/wn10-2/wn10-202.html, you would use acid-free paper around photos. To store paper that has a high acid content, put the papers in folders and storage boxes with an alkaline reserve to prevent acid migration. Interleave your papers with sheets of alkaline-buffered paper.

The buffered paper protects your item from acids that move from areas of high to areas of low concentration. Buffers neutralize acids in paper. A buffer is an alkaline chemical such as calcium carbonate. So you have the choice to use the buffered or non-buffered paper depending on whether your photos are stored against other acid-free materials or printed on acid-free paper.

Photos:

Interweave photos with waxed paper or polyester web covered blotters. Store photos away from overhead water pipes in a cool, dry area with stable humidity and temperatures, not in attics or basements. Keep photos out of direct sunlight and fluorescent lights when on display. Color slides have their own storage requirements.

Keep photos from touching rubber bands, cellophane tape, rubber cement, or paper clips. Poor quality photo paper and paper used in most envelopes and album sleeves also cause photos to deteriorate. Instead, store photos in chemically stable plastic made of polyester, polypropylene, triacetate, or polyethylene. Don't use PCV or vinyl sleeves. Plastic enclosures preserve photos best and keep out the fingerprints and scratches.

Albumen prints are interleaved between groups of photographs. Matte and glossy collodion prints should not be touched by bare hands. Store the same as albumen prints—interleaved between groups of photos. Silver gelatin printing and developing photo papers are packed in plastic bags inside plastic boxes. Carbon prints and Woodbury prints are packed horizontally. Photomechanical prints are interleaved every two inches and packed in boxes. Transport color photos horizontally—face up.

Chromogenic prints and negatives are packed in plastic bags inside boxes. If you're dealing with cased photos, pack the ambrotypes and pannotypes horizontally in padded containers. Cover the glass of Daguerreotype photos and pack horizontally in padded containers.

Pollutants from the air trapped inside holders and folders destroy photos and paper. Use buffered enclosures for black and white prints and negatives. Use non-buffered paper enclosures to store color prints and color print negatives or cyanotypes and albumen prints.

Store your tintypes horizontally. If you have collodion glass plate negatives, use supports for the glass and binders, and pack horizontally in padded containers. The surface texture of photos stored in plastic can deteriorate. It's called ferrotyping. So don't store negatives in plastic. If you store your photos in paper enclosures, be aware that paper is porous. Instead of plastic or paper storage, put photos in **glass plate negative sleeves in acid-free non-buffered enclosures**.

Then store vertically between pieces of foam board. Where do you find glass plate negative sleeves that can be stored in acid-free non-buffered enclosures? Buy storage materials from companies catering to conservationists, such as *Light Impressions ®*. They're the leading resource for archival supplies. Also look in local craft stores.

Talk to your state archives conservation specialist. Some documents require the work of a trained conservationist. Before you sterilize mold away with bleach, ask your state archives conservationist whether the bleach will ruin your diary or heirloom.

Photo Albums:

Don't make or buy photo albums with "peel-back" plastic over sticky cardboard pieces because they are chemically unstable and could damage anything stored there. Instead, use photo-packet pages made from chemically stable plastic made of polyester, polypropylene, triacetate, or polyethylene. An excellent album would contain archival-quality pages using polyester mounting corners. Acid-free paper mounting corners are next best.

Vellum or Parchment Documents:

Interleave between folders, and pack oversize materials flat. If you have prints and drawings made from chemically stable media, then interleave between folders and pack in cartons. Oversize prints and drawings should be packed in bread trays, or map drawers, placed on poly-covered plywood. Be careful the mildew from plywood doesn't paste onto the back of your print. Look at the poly-covering on the wood.

Take off the frames of your drawings or prints if you can. Books with leather and vellum bindings need to be packed spine down in crates one layer deep. Books and pamphlets should be separated with freezer paper and always packed spine down in crates one layer deep.

Bread trays work well to store parchment and vellum manuscripts that are interleaved between folders. Anything oversize gets packed flat. Posters need to be packed in containers lined with garbage bags because they are *coated* papers. Watercolors and hand-colored prints or inks should be interleaved between folders and packed in crates. Paintings need to be stored *face up* without touching the paint layer. Carry them horizontally.

Computer Tapes and Disks, Audio and Video Tapes:

Store those 'dinosaur' computer tapes in plastic bags packed vertically with plenty of room. Store tapes in plastic crates away from light, heat, or cold. Never touch the magnetic media. If you have an open reel tape, pick up by the hub or reel. Floppy disks should be packed vertically in plastic bags and stored in plastic crates.

With DVDs and CDs, pack vertically in plastic crates and store in plastic drawers or cardboard cartons. Careful—don't touch or scratch the recordable surface. Handle the CD or DVD by the edge. Place audio and video tapes vertically in plastic holders and store them in plastic crates.

Disks made of shellac or acetate and vinyl disks are held by their edges and packed vertically in ethafoam-padded crates. Make sure nothing heavy is placed on CDs, DVDs, tapes, or other disks. You can find ethafoam in most craft stores, or order from a company specializing in storage or presentation tools such as Light Impressions ®.

◆   ◆   ◆

Resources:
American Institute for Conservation
1717 K Street, NW, Suite 200
Washington, DC 20006
tel: 202-452-9545
fax: 202-452-9328
email: info@aic-faic.org
website: http://aic.stanford.edu

Light Impressions (Archival Supplies)
PO Box 22708
Rochester, NY 14692-2708
1-800-828-6216
http://www.lightimpressionsdirect.com

Bibliography:

WAAC Newsletter
http://palimpsest.stanford.edu/aic'disaster

WAAC Newsletter, Vol. 19, No 2 (May, 1997) articles and charts online by Betty Walsh, Conservator, BC Archives, Canada and the Walsh's information at: http://palimpsest.stanford.edu/waac/wn/wn10/wn10-2/wn10-202.html. The site contains material from the WAAC Newsletter, Volume 10, Number 2, May 1988, pp.2-5.

Curatorial Care of Works of Art on Paper, New York: Intermuseum Conservation Association, 1987.

Library Materials Preservation Manual: Practical Methods for Preserving Books, Pamphlets, and Other Printed Materials, Heidi Kyle. 1984

Archives & Manuscripts: Conservation—A Manual on Physical Care and Management, Mary Lynn Ritzenthaler, Society of American Archivists: Chicago, 1993.

10

Personal or Medical Histories as Points of View within Social Histories

Autobiographies, biographies, personal histories, plays, and monologues present a point of view. Are all sides given equal emphasis? Will the audience choose favorite characters? Cameras give fragments, points of view, and bits and pieces. Viewers will see what the videographer or photographer intends to be seen. The interviewee will also be trying to put his point of view across and tell the story from his perspective.

Will the photographer or videographer be in agreement with the interviewee? Or if you are recording for print transcript, will your point of view agree with the interviewee's perspective and experience if your basic 'premise,' where you two are coming from, are not in agreement? Think this over as you write your list of questions. Do both of you agree on your central issue on which you'll focus for the interview?

How are you going to turn spoken words into text for your paper hard copy transcript? Will you transcribe verbatim, correct the grammar, or quote as you hear the spoken words? Oral historians really need to transcribe the exact spoken word. You can leave out the 'ahs' and 'oms' or loud pauses, as the interviewee thinks what to say next. You don't want to sound like a court reporter, but you do want to have an accurate record transcribed of what was spoken.

You're also not editing for a movie, unless you have permission to turn the oral history into a TV broadcast, where a lot gets cut out of the interview for time constraints. For that, you'd need written permission so words won't be taken out of context and strung together in the editing room to say something different from what the interviewee intended to say.

Someone talking could put in wrong names, forget what they wanted to say, or repeat themselves. They could mumble, ramble, or do almost anything. So you would have to sit down and weed out redundancy when you can or decide on presenting exactly what you've heard as transcript.

When someone reads the transcript in text, they won't have what you had in front of you, and they didn't see and hear the live presentation or the videotape. It's possible to misinterpret gestures or how something is spoken, the mood or tone, when reading a text transcript. Examine all your sources. Use an ice-breaker to get someone talking.

If a woman is talking about female-interest issues, she may feel more comfortable talking to another woman. Find out whether the interviewee is more comfortable speaking to someone of his or her own age. Some older persons feel they can relate better to someone close to their own age than someone in high school, but it varies. Sometimes older people can speak more freely to a teenager.

The interviewee must be able to feel comfortable with the interviewer and know he or she will not be judged. Sometimes it helps if the interviewer is the same ethnic group or there is someone present of the same group or if new to the language, a translator is present.

Read some books on oral history field techniques. Read the National Genealogical Society Quarterly (NGSQ). Also look at The American Genealogist (TAG), The Genealogist, and The New England Historical and Genealogical Register (The Register). If you don't know the maiden name of say, your grandmother's mother, and no relative knows either because it wasn't on her death certificate, try to reconstruct the lives of the males who had ever met the woman whose maiden name is unknown.

Maybe she did business with someone before marriage or went to school or court. Someone may have recorded the person's maiden name before her marriage. Try medical records if any were kept. There was no way to find my mother's grandmother's maiden name until I started searching to see whether she had any brothers in this country. She had to have come as a passenger on a ship around 1880 as she bought a farm. Did her husband come with her?

Was the farm in his name? How many brothers did she have in this country with her maiden surname? If the brothers were not in this country, what countries did they come from and what cities did they live in before they bought the farm in Albany? If I could find out what my great grandmother's maiden name was through any brothers living at the time, I could contact their descendants perhaps and see whether any male or female lines are still in this country or where else on the globe.

Perhaps a list of midwives in the village at the time is recorded in a church or training school for midwives. Fix the person in time and place. Find out whom she might have done business with and whether any records of that business exist. What businesses did she patronize? Look for divorce or court records, change of name records, and other legal documents.

Look at local sources. Did anyone save records from bills of sale for weddings, purchases of homes, furniture, debutante parties, infant supplies, or even medical records? Look at nurses' licenses, midwives' registers, employment contracts, and teachers' contracts, alumni associations for various schools, passports, passenger lists, alien registration cards, naturalization records, immigrant aid societies, city directories, and cross-references.

Try religious and women's clubs, lineage and village societies, girl scouts and similar groups, orphanages, sanatoriums, hospitals, police records. Years ago there was even a Eugenics Record Office. What about the women's prisons? The first one opened in 1839—Mount Pleasant Female Prison, NY.

Try voters' lists. If your relative is from another country, try records in those villages or cities abroad. Who kept the person's diaries? Have you checked the Orphan Train records? Try ethnic and religious societies and genealogy associations for that country. Most ethnic genealogy societies have a special interest group for even the smallest villages in various countries.

You can start one and put up a Web site for people who also come from there in past centuries. Check alimony, divorce, and court records, widow's pensions of veterans, adoptions, orphanages, foster homes, medical records, birth, marriage, and death certificates, social security, immigration, pet license owners' files, prisons, alumni groups from schools, passenger lists, military, and other legal records.

When all historical records are being tied together, you can add the DNA testing to link all those cousins. Check military pensions on microfilms in the National Archives. See the bibliography section of this book for further resources on highly recommended books and articles on oral history field techniques and similar historical subjects.

Preparing Personal or Medical and Family History Time Capsules for a Journey

Be personal in a personal history life story. The more personal you are, the more eternal is your life story. More people will view or read it again and again far into the future. You can emphasize your life's journey and look at the world through your own eyes. To make the structure salable, 'meander' your life as you would travel on a journey. Perhaps you're a winding river meandering around obstacles and competitors. At each stop, you learn your own capabilities and your own place in the world.

The more you meander, the more you take away the urgency from your story that sets up tension in the audience and keeps them on the edge of their seat. Don't let the meandering overpower your sense of urgency. Don't dwell on your reaction. Focus on your action to people and situations. Stay active in your own personal history. In other words, don't repeat how you reacted, but show how you acted.

Before you sit down to write your autobiography, think of yourself in terms of going on a journey inside the privacy of your purse or wallet. May your purse is the only place where you really do have any privacy. Come up for air when you have hit bottom. Bob up to the sunshine, completely changed or at least matured.

If you have really grown, you will not be blinded by the light, in the figurative sense, as the song goes. Instead, the light gives you insight. So now you have vision along with some hindsight. The next step is learning how to promote and market your salable personal history or life story.

A biography reports the selected events of another person's life—usually 12 major events in the six various significant events also known as "turning points" and also known as "transition points" of life that would include the highlights of significant events for each of the six stages of growth: 1) infanthood, 2) childhood, 3) teen years 4) young adulthood 5) middle life 6) maturity.

Selling Ghostwritten or Journalistic Life Stories

Launch your salable life story in the major national press and in various newspapers and magazines of niche markets related to the events in your life, such as weekly newspapers catering to a group: senior citizens, your ethnic group, your local area, or your occupation or area of interest. Your personal history time capsule may be saved to disk and also uploaded to the Web. What about looking for movie deals and book publishers?

If you don't have the money to produce your autobiography as a video biography, or even a film or commercial movie, or publish it for far less cost as a print-on-demand published book, you may wish to find a co-production partner to finance the production of your life story as a cinematic film or made-for-TV video.

At the same time you could contact literary agents and publishers, but one front-page article in a national newspaper or daily newspaper can do wonders to move your life story in front of the gaze of publishers and producers. While you're waiting for a reporter to pay attention to the news angle you have selected for your life story, I highly recommend Michael Wiese's book <u>Film and Video Marketing</u> because it lists some co-production partners as the following:

Private Investors/Consortiums

Foreign Governments (blocked funds)

Financiers
Corporations
Theatrical Distributors
International Theatrical Distributors
International Sales Agents
Home Video
International Home Video
Pay TV
Syndicators
Record Companies
Music Publishers
Book Publishers
Toy Companies
Licensing and Merchandising Firms
Sponsors (products, services)
Public Relations Firms
Marketing Companies/Consultants
Film Bookers

You can also contact actors, directors, producers, feature distributors, home video distributors, entertainment lawyers, brokers, accountants, animation houses, production houses, video post production houses, labs, film facilities, and agents with your script and ask the owners whether they'd be interested in bartering budget items, deferring, or investing in your script.

Private investors could also be professional investors, venture capitalists, and even doctors and dentists who may wish to finance a movie if the potential interests them. You can sell points in your film to investors who finance it as a group of investors, each buying a small percentage of the film for an investment fee.

Or you can approach film investment corporations that specialize in investing in and producing films as partners. They are publicized or listed in the entertainment trade magazines going to producers and workers in the entertainment and film or video industry.

You market your script not only to agents and producers, but to feature distributors, film financiers and co-production partners. This is the first step in finding a way to take your autobiography from script to screen. Learn who distributes what before you approach anyone.

If you want to approach video instead of film, you might wish to know that children's video programming is the fastest-growing genre in original programming. Children's titles account for 10%-15% of the overall home video revenues.

According to one of Michael Wiese's books written in the nineties, *Home Video: Producing For The Home Market*, "With retail prices falling and alternative retail outlets expanding, children's programming will soon become one of the most profitable segments of the video market." He was right.

What has happened in the new millennium is that children's program is doing wonderfully. Why? Children's video is repeatable. Children watch the same tape 30 to 50 times. Children's video sells for comparatively lower prices than feature films.

Children's video also rents well. Children's tapes sell it toy stores, book stores, children's stores, and in stores like Woolworth's and Child World. Manufacturers sell tapes at Toy Fair and the American Booksellers Association conventions.

For these reasons, you may wish to write your autobiography as a script for children's video or as a children's book. Video is a burgeoning industry.

According to the market research firm, Fairfield Group, in 1985, the prerecorded video business earned $ 3.3 billion in sales and rentals. This nearly equaled the record and theatrical box office revenues for the same year. The world VCR population is about 100 million. Today we have the DVD and the Internet streaming video.

Back in 1985, the U.S. and Japan accounted for half of the VCRs, followed by the United Kingdom, (9 million) West Germany (nearly 7 million), and Canada, Australia, Turkey, and France (about 3 million each). Spain reported 2 million VCRs. By 1991, the number of VCR ownership increased as prices slowly came down.

Today, in the 21st century, the prerecorded video business has quickly moved to DVD disks, downloadable at a price Internet-based movies, and video tapes are on the way to being a memory of the eighties and early nineties. In the next decade, another media format will be in fashion to replace videos on DVDs and streaming Internet video. The idea is to keep transferring the story from one form of technology to another so that videos made today will be able to be viewed by people in the next century.

The European VCR markets grew faster than in the U.S. during the eighties and nineties just as the DVD markets grew in the early 21st century because there were fewer entertainment alternatives—fewer TV stations, restricted viewing hours, fewer pay TV services, and fewer movie theatres.

You should not overlook the foreign producers for your script. Include Canadian cable TV, foreign agents, and foreign feature film and video producers among your contacts. Most university libraries open to the public for research include directories listing foreign producers. Photocopy their addresses and send them a query letter and one-page synopsis of your script. Don't overlook the producers from non-English speaking countries. Your script can be translated or dubbed.

You might attend film market type conventions and conferences. They draw producers from a variety of countries. In 1989 at the former Cinetex Film Market in Las Vegas, producers from Canada, Italy, Israel, Spain, and other foreign countries sat next to script writers. All of them were receptive to receiving scripts. They handed one another their business cards. You can learn a lot at summer film markets and film festivals about what kind of scripts are in demand.

Keep a list of which film markets will meet. In the U.S. there are 3 to 5 film markets a year and many more film festivals. Seek out the foreign and local producers with track records and see whether they'd be interested in your script if you have a life story in the form of a script, treatment, or story. Perhaps your theme has some relation to a producer's country or ethnic group. Lots of films are made in Asia, in the Middle East (Israel, Egypt and Tunisia), in Latin America, and Europe or Canada.

Seek out the Australian producers also and New Zealand or India. If you have a low-budget film or home video script set in Korea, Philippines, Japan, or Taiwan, or a specialty film such as Karate or something that appeals to the Indian film market, contact those producers and script agents in those countries. Find out the budget limitations that producers have in the different countries.

Social issues documentaries based on your autobiography are another market for home video. Vestron and other home video distributors use hard-hitting documentaries. Collecting documentary video tapes is like collecting copies of National Geographic magazine. You never throw them out. Tapes are also sold by direct mail. Companies producing and distributing documentaries include MCA, MGM/UA, Vestron, Victory, CBS/Fox, Warner, Media, Karl, Monterey, Thorn/EMI, Embassy, and USA, to name a few.

If you write your autobiography or another's biography as a romance, you might wish to write a script for the video romance series market. Romance video has its roots in the paperback novel. However, the biggest publishers of medical, gene hunter, scientist, and nurse-type romance novels have little recognition in retail video stores.

Among consumers, yes; wholesalers and retailers, no. Bookstores, yes. The problem is with pricing. To sell romance videos in bookstores, the tapes would have to be sold at less than $29. In video stores, they can be positioned the same as $59 feature films on video.

Production costs to make high quality romance videos are high. Top stars, top writers, hit book titles, exotic locations, music and special effects are required. Huge volumes of tapes must be sold to break even. Then producers have to search for pay TV, broadcast, or foreign partners. The budget for a one-hour video tape of a thin romance story comes to $500,000.

It's far better to make a low-budget feature film. Romance as a genre has never previously appealed to the video retail buyer. In contrast, a romance paperback sells for a few dollars. Now the question remains: Would women buy a romance-genre video DVD priced at $9.95?

Romance novels successfully have been adapted to audio tape for listening at far less than the cost of video. There is a market for audio scripts of short romance novels and novellas. What is becoming popular today are videos and 'movies' downloadable from the Internet that you can watch on your computer screen or save to a DVD since DVD burners became affordable and popular. Try adapting highlights of your romance or life story novel to a play, skit, or monologue.

The only way romance videos would work is by putting together a multi-partnered structure that combines pay TV, home video, book publishing, and domestic and foreign TV. In the eighties, was anyone doing romance video tapes? Yes. Prism Video produced six feature-length romance films, acquired from Comworld. In 1985 the tapes sold for $11.95.

Comworld had limited TV syndication exposure and was one of the first to come out with romance videos. Karl/Lorimar came out with eight romance films from L/A House Productions on a budget of $400,000 each. They were also priced at $11.95 in 1985. To break even, a company has to sell about 60,000 units per title.

Twenty years later, think about adapting to a play the romance DVD video and the downloadable Internet video. What's available to adapt as educational material? Write for various age groups on niche subjects that would appeal to teachers. Follow their rules on what is appropriate for their classrooms. The market also is open for stage and radio/Internet broadcast skits and plays geared to older adults as performers and audiences.

Other media are like open doors to finding a way to put your life story on a disk. Any interview, script, or story can go from print-on-demand published novel or true story book to radio script or stage play. A video can move from a digital high 8 camcorder with a Firewire 1394 cable attached to a personal computer rapidly into the hard disk drive via Windows XP Movie Maker software. Or you can purchase the latest camcorders that record directly onto a mini-disk that looks similar to a small CD or DVD and which can be played directly on your CD or DVD player or saved and played in your computer.

From there it can be saved as a WMV file (a Windows Media file). Then the file can be recorded on a DVD, if long, or a CD if under one hour. Poems can be written, read, and 'burned' to a compact disk (CD) and then mailed out as greeting cards, love letters, or personal histories. Short videos can be emailed.

Romance or life story highlights novels and scripts on audio tape cost less to produce. This market occasionally advertises for romantic novel manuscripts, scripts, and stories in a variety of writer's magazines.

Check out the needs of various magazines for journalists and writers online. If you read a lot of romance genre novels or write in this style, you may want to write your autobiography in this genre, but you'd have to market to publishers who use this genre or biographies in other genres such as factual biography.

If your autobiography is set on events which occurred in your childhood, you might prefer to concentrate on writing appropriate for children's video programming. It's a lot easier to sell to the producers who are basking in the current explosion of children's video programming. Perhaps it's your mission to use the video format to teach children.

Will the script of your medical-oriented case history, life experience, or personal history do the following?

teach,
mentor,
motivate,
inspire,
or inform viewers who can be:
children,
teenagers,
parents
or midlifers on their quests for self-identify:
or in their search for facts:
to use as guidelines in making their own decisions:
about life's journeys and writing an introspective journal?

Can your diary be dynamic, dramatic, and empowering to others who may be going through similar stages of life? Are your characters charismatic and memorable, likable and strong?

A medical or genetic case history, personal history, life story or autobiography when videotaped or filed as a feature-length movie can spring out of a diary or an inner personal journal (which dialogues with the people who impact your life and observes selected, important events). Write medicate and personal history reports for time capsule and include individual DNA reports. The goal is for family members to pass these time capsules onto members of the next generation.

They should be able to be copied for each family member. Time capsules could contain in addition to medical histories and DNA reports, family histories, keepsake albums, and any audio or video recordings as well as photographs, diaries, and text of numerous generations. Put them in several formats so that when technology evolves, the materials can be copied and transferred to the next level of technology. Medical writers also can be personal historians.

◆   ◆   ◆

Medical Writing or Ghostwriting about Pets: Care, Food, Travel, Adventures, History, Genes, and Controversial Issues in the News—Consumer Surveillance and Pet Cloning

There's another branch of nutritional genomics that instead of only testing your DNA to find out which foods are healthiest for your genes, focuses on *manipulating plant micronutrients* to improve human health. See the article on the Internet, a PDF file on a Web site at: **http://www.ipef.br/melhoramento/genoma/pdfs/dellapenna99.pdf**.

The volume of imported food is growing each year. Consumers have a field cut out for them—surveillance. As FDA increases its examinations and sampling at borders, consumers can work together to research information about food imports and inspection.

A laboratory can only sample so many products. Consumers can take a role in food security, perhaps looking at industry to identify problems or threats. What the consumer's role entails is better information and collaboration. Everyone needs to keep costs down.

Plant biotechnology of food and feed is another area of consumer interest. If you buy food that comes from overseas, do you ever wonder who oversees the packaging and shipping of those products? Are there really enough inspectors to go around? Consumers worry about the widespread use of sugar in soft drinks. In addition to having your DNA tested, you need to understand how what you eat influences your health at all ages.

Another way consumers can oversee quality control is by forming public interest research groups funded by grant money, private donors, institutions, or the government. You can become a volunteer in nutritional genomics, an ombudsman, a lobbyist, or start your own consumer research interest group.

You can turn a hobby of medical ghostwriting, nutritional genomics or DNA for ancestry and genealogy into a business by affiliating yourself with a university lab which you contract to do testing from your DNA testing clients. There are open doors for consumer involvement depending upon your skills and interests. Nutritional genomics needs public speakers and technical writers to relay to the public what innovations the experts are bringing to healthcare and food systems design.

From running a summer camp for teens interested in nutritional genomics internships or learning experiences to recruiting DNA donors to create a DNA bank or in researching and writing about genomics, there are a variety of doors. Consumers have power in numbers. You can even enter as a venture capitalist with a goal of raising funds even if you have no funds of your own and plenty of determination to learn to ropes.

Don't overlook nutritional genomics for the pet care industry from foods to medicine. Contact the veterinary schools about their research on how foods affect genetic signatures of pets or race horses. Check out the Web site for Research Diets at: http://www.researchdiets.com/.

Research Diets, a New Jersey company since 1984 has formulated more than 6,000 distinct *laboratory* animal diets for research in all areas of biology and related fields at hundreds of pharmaceutical, university, and government laboratories around the world. Nutritional genomics isn't only for humans or laboratory animals. Did you ever think about how your dog or cat could benefit by genetic testing to determine which foods are healthiest?

Talk to your veterinarian to see who is researching how nutraceuticals and better food can help your pet's health, especially when the pet is older. What about nutritional genomics for farm animals or pets? Find out who is doing what kind of nutrition research for better health.

Appendix A

Associations of Interest to Medical or Science Journalists and Ghostwriters

American Dietetic Association
http://www.eatright.org

American Obesity Association
http://www.obesity.org

American Society for Nutritional Sciences
http://www.asns.org/

American Society for Clinical Nutrition
http://www.ascn.org/

The Annapolis Center for Science-Based Public Policy
http://www.annapoliscenter.org

Association of Food & Drug Officials
http://www.afdo.org

American Diabetes Association
http://www.diabetes.org

American Farm Bureau Federation
http://www.fb.com

American Heart Association
http://www.americanheart.org

Botanical Center for Age-Related Diseases
http://nccam.nih.gov/news/2005/040705.htm

Calorie Control Council
http://www.caloriecontrol.org

Center for Health Promotion
http://pan.ilsi.org

Consumer Healthcare Products Association
http://www.caloriecontrol.org

CropLife America
http://www.croplifeamerica.org

Egg Nutrition Center
http://www.enc-online.org

Food Marketing Institute
http://www.fmi.org

Food Allergy Research and Resource Program
http://www.farrp.org

Grocery Manufacturers of America
http://www.gmabrands.com

International Association for Food Protection
http://www.foodprotection.org

National Dairy Council/Dairy Management
http://www.dairyinfo.com

National Policy and Resource Center on Nutrition and Aging
http://www.fiu.edu/~nutreldr

North American Agricultural Journalists
http://naaj.tamu.edu/

Society for Nutrition Education
http://www.sne.org

World Sugar Research Organization
http://www.wsro.org

Government-Related Agencies

Centers for Disease Control and Prevention
http://www.cdc.gov

Center for Food Safety and Applied Nutrition
http://www.crfsan.fda.gov

Fight BAC ™
http://www.fightbck.org

Food and Drug Administration: Consumer Inquiries
http://www.fda.gov

Joint Institute for Food Safety and Applied Nutrition
http://www.jifsan.umd.edu

National Cancer Institute: Press Office
http://www.nci.nih.gov

National Digestive Disease Information Clearinghouse
http://www.niddk.nih.gov

National Diabetes Information Clearinghouse
http://www.niddk.ninh.gov

National Health Information Center
http://health.gov/NHIC

National Institutes of Health
http://www.nih.gov

National Marine Fisheries Service
http://www.nmfs.noaa.gov

President's Council on Physical Fitness and Sports
http://fitness.gov

US Dept. of Agriculture
http://www.usda.gov

USDA/Food, Nutrition, and Consumer Services
http://www.fns.usda.gov/fncs

USDA/ Food Safety and Inspection Service Information
http://www.fsis.usda.gov

USDA/Meat and Poultry Hotline
http://www.fsis.usda.gov/Home/index.asp

USDA/Animal and Plant Health Inspection Service
http://www.aphis.usda.gov

USDA/Foreign Agricultural Service
http://www.fas.usda.gov

USDA/National Agricultural Library
http://www.nalusda.gov

USDA/National Agriculture Statistics Service
http://www.fas.usda.gov

US Department of Health and Human Services
http://www.hhs.gov

Foodborne Illness Education Information Center
http://www.nalusda.gov/foodborne/index.html

US Department of Health and Human Services
http://www.hhs.gov

US Environmental Protection Agency
http://www.epa.gov

US Federal Trade Commission
http://www.ftc.gov

◆   ◆   ◆

Associations of Interest to Medical or Science Journalists and Ghostwriters

American Medical Writers Association
40 West Gude Drive, Suite 101
Rockville, MD 20850-1192
http://www.amwa.org/default.asp?ID=1

American Society of Indexers (for indexing careers)
10200 West 44th Avenue, Suite 304,
Wheat Ridge, CO 80033
http://www.asindexing.org/site/index.html

American Society of Journalists and Authors
1501 Broadway, Suite 302
New York, NY 10036
http://www.asja.org

Association of Health Care Journalists (AHCJ)
Center for Excellence in Health Care Journalism
Missouri School of Journalism
10 Neff Hall
Columbia, MO 62511
http://www.ahcj.umn.edu/

Association of Professional Writing Consultants
http://www.consultingsuccess.org/index.htm

Council of Biology Editors
http://www.monroecc.edu/depts/library/cbe.htm

Council of the Advancement of Science Writing
P.O. Box 910
Hedgesville, WV 25427
http://www.casw.org/
Careers in Science Writing:
http://www.casw.org/careers.htm

Education Writers Association
2122 P Street, NW Suite 201
Washington, DC 20037
http://www.ewa.org/

International Food, Wine & Travel Writers Association (IFW&TWA)
1142 South Diamond Bar Boulevard #177
Diamond Bar, CA 91765-2203
http://www.ifwtwa.org/index.html
Journalism.org—Researches, Resources & Ideas to Improve Journalism
http://www.journalism.org/
National Association of
Science Writers, Inc.
P.O. Box 890, Hedgesville, WV 25427
http://www.nasw.org/

North American Agricultural Journalists
http://naaj.tamu.edu/

Society of Professional Journalists
Eugene S. Pulliam National Journalism Center
3909 N. Meridian St., Indianapolis, IN 46208
http://www.spj.org/

Society for Technical Communication
http://www.stc.org/

Text and Academic Authors Association
TAA
P.O. Box 76477
St. Petersburg, FL
http://www.taaonline.net/

World Association of Medical Editors
http://www.wame.org/
http://www.wame.org/index.htm

Diversified Media Associations of Interest to all Communicators

American Business Press
http://www.americanbusinesspress.com/

American Society of Business Press Editors
http://www.asbpe.org/

Associated Business Writers of America
http://www.poewar.com/articles/associations.htm

Associazioni ed Enti Professionali-America
http://www.alice.it/writers/grp.wri/wgrpame.htm
Contains a list of South American, Canadian, and US writers' organizations, including language translation firms.

American Marketing Association
http://www.marketingpower.com/content1539.php

Association of Professional Communications Consultants
http://www.consultingsuccess.org/index.htm

Writer's Encyclopedia A-Z List
WritersMarket.com
http://www.writersmarket.com/encyc/azlist.asp

Editorial Freelancers Association
http://www.the-efa.org/

Editor's Guild
http://www.edsguild.org/become.htm

The current online Yellow Pages, published annually since 1997 includes listings by skills as well as a specialties index. This association published the hardcopy, Yellow Pages, a listing of Association members who wished to advertise their skills and specialties, between 1989 and 1999.

http://www.tiac.net/users/freelanc/YP.html

International Women's Writing Guild
http://www.iwwg.com/index.php, Or: http://www.iwwg.com

The International Women's Writing Guild, headquartered in New York and founded in 1976, is a network for the personal and professional empowerment of women through writing.

Video Software Dealers Association
http://www.vsda.org/Resource.phx/vsda/index.htx
Public Relations Society of America
http://www.prsa.org/
Deep Dish TV
http://www.deepdishtv.org/pages/catalogue13.htm
Video History Project
http://www.experimentaltvcenter.org/history/groups/gtext.php3?id=37
Advertising Research Foundation
http://www.arfsite.org/
The Mail Preference Service
http://www.dmaconsumers.org/offmailinglist.html
Advertising Associations Directory
http://paintedcows.com/associations.html
Mailing Fulfillment Service Association
http://www.mfsanet.org/pages/index.cfm?pageid=1
Television Bureau of Advertising
http://www.tvb.org/nav/build_frameset.asp?url=/docs/homepage.asp
Home Improvement Research Institute

http://www.hiri.org/abouthiri.htm
Writers-Editors Network
http://www.writers-editors.com/
Professional and Technical Consultants Association
http://www.patca.org/html/articles/ratesurvey/ratesurvey1.htm
Association of Independent Commercial Producers
http://www.aicp.com/splash-noswf.html
National Cable & Telecommunications Association
http://www.ncta.com/
International Association of Women in Radio and Television
http://www.iawrt.org/
National Communication Association
http://www.natcom.org/nca/Template2.asp
The Association for Women in Communications
http://www.womcom.org/
Society of Telecommunications Consultants
http://www.stcconsultants.org/
European Training Media Association
http://www.etma.org/
Advertising Research Foundation
641 Lexington Avenue • New York, NY 10022
http://www.arfsite.org/
International Women's Media Foundation
http://www.iwmf.org/training/womensmedia.php

Independent Publishers Group
http://www.ipgbook.com/index.cfm?userid=36155756
American Society of Media Photographers
150 North Second Street, Philadelphia, PA 19106
(Electronic imaging and digital technology)
http://www.asmp.org/
International Interactive Communications Society
http://users.rcn.com/sfiics/
International Multimedia Association
http://www.emmac.org/
National Cable Television Association
http://www.museum.tv/archives/etv/N/htmlN/nationalcabl/
nationalcabl.htm

Information Technology Association of America
http://www.itaa.org/eweb/StartPage.aspx

Personal and Oral History Associations

Association of Personal Historians
http://www.personalhistorians.org/index.html

Oral History Association
http://omega.dickinson.edu/organizations/oha/about.html

International Oral History Association
http://www.ioha.fgv.br/ioha/english/index.html

Texas Oral History Association
http://www.baylor.edu/TOHA/

Southwest Oral History Association
http://soha.fullerton.edu/

New England Association for Oral History
http://www.ucc.uconn.edu/~cohadm01/neaoh.html

Michigan Oral History Association
http://www.umich.edu/pres/history/oral.html

UCLA Oral History Program
http://www.library.ucla.edu/libraries/special/ohp/ohpindex.htm

"California As I Saw It," First Person Narratives of California's Early Years: 1849-1900. The Library of Congress.
http://memory.loc.gov/ammem/cbhtml/cbhome.html

Nutrition and Health-Related Associations, Research Institutes, Corporations, Academies, and University Programs

American Academy of Family Physicians: http://www.aafp.org/
American Association of Family and Consumer Sciences: http://www.aafcs.org/
American Dietetic Association: http://www.eatright.org/

American Heart Association: http://www.americanheart.org/
American Institute for Cancer Research: http://www.aicr.org/
American Public Health Association: http://www.apha.org/
American Society of Clinical Nutrition: http://www.ascn.org/
Center for Science in the Public Interest: http://www.cspinet.org/
Chocolate Manufacturers Association: http://www.chocolateusa.org/
Consumer Federation of America: http://www.consumerfed.org/
Consumer Healthcare Products Association: http://www.chpa-info.org/
Council for Responsible Nutrition: http://www.crnusa.org/
Egg Nutrition Center: http://www.enc-online.org/
Federal Trade Commission: http://www.ftc.gov/
Food and Nutrition Board, Institute of Medicine: http://www.iom.edu/board.asp?id=3788
Foundation for American Communications: http://www.facsnet.org/
Asian Food Information Center: http://www.afic.org/Press%20Centre.htm
Institute of Food Technologists: http://www.ift.org/cms/
International Dairy Foods Association: http://www.idfa.org/
International Life Sciences Institute: http://www.ilsi.org/
Kleinfeld Kaplan & Becker: http://www.fda.gov/ohrms/dockets/dailys/00/Aug00/082400/cp0001.pdf
Lehigh University, Department of Journalism and Communication: http://www.lehigh.edu/~injrl/sciwrit/
National Cancer Institute, US National Institutes of Health: http://www.cancer.gov/
National Cooperative Business Association: http://www.ncba.coop/
National Food Processors Association: http://www.worldfooddayusa.org/CMS/2951/8939.aspx
National Potato Promotion Board: http://www.uspotatoes.com/
Office of Dietary Supplements, National Institutes of Health: http://ods.od.nih.gov/
The Popcorn Board: http://www.popcorn.org/index.cfm
Purdue University, National Institutes of Health Botanicals Center for Age-Related Diseases: http://www.purdue.edu/UNS/html4ever/000920.Weaver.nihcenter.html
Purdue University, Department of Foods and Nutrition: http://www.cfs.purdue.edu/
Rutgers University, Nutraceuticals Institute: http://foodsci.rutgers.edu/nci/
Soyfoods Association of North America: http://www.soyfoods.org/

Saint Joseph's University, Erivan K. Haub School of Business: http://www.sju.edu/

Tufts School of Medicine and Nutrition: http://www.tufts.edu/med/nutrition-infection/

Tufts University Health and Nutrition Letter: http://healthletter.tufts.edu/

United Soybean Board: http://www.unitedsoybean.org/

United States Department of Agriculture, Agricultural Research Service: http://www.ars.usda.gov/main/main.htm

United States Food and Drug Administration, Center for Food Safety and Applied Nutrition: http://www.cfsan.fda.gov/list.html

University of California, Davis: http://www.ucdavis.edu/index.html

University of California, Davis, California Institute of Food and Agricultural Research: http://aic.ucdavis.edu/

University of California, Davis, Robert Mondavi Institute for Wine and Food Science: http://www.news.ucdavis.edu/mondavi/iwfs_facts.html

University of Illinois, Department of Food Science and Human Nutrition: http://www.fshn.uiuc.edu/

University of Illinois, Functional Foods for Health Program: http://www.ag.uiuc.edu/~ffh/ffh.html

University of Massachusetts, Department of Food Science: http://www.umass.edu/foodsci/

University of Missouri, Columbia, Department of Food Science and Human Nutrition: http://outreach.missouri.edu/hes/food.htm

University of Missouri, Columbia, Missouri School of Journalism: http://journalism.missouri.edu/

University of Southern California, School of Pharmacy: http://www.usc.edu/schools/pharmacy/

Virginia Tech Center for Food and Nutrition Policy: http://www.vt.edu/

Food Safety Research Information Office: http://www.nal.usda.gov/fsrio/acad.htm

APPENDIX B

Medical Writing and Ghostwriting Bibliography

Reprinted here, courtesy of and with the permission of the American Medical Writers Association-Delaware Valley Chapter that prepared this Bibliography. See this information and more at the American Medical Writers Association's, Delaware Valley Chapter's Web site at: http://www.amwa-dvc.org/toolkit/index.shtml#1a

Books

Style Guides
American Medical Association Manual of Style, 9th edition. Baltimore, MD et al.: Williams & Wilkins, 1998. Contact information: www.wwilkins.com, 800-638-0672.

Medical English Usage and Abusage. Edith Schwager (AMWA member), Phoenix, AZ, Oryx Press, 1991. Contact information: www.greenwood.com, 800-225-5800.

Mathematics into Type, Ellen Swanson, American Mathematical Society, Providence, RI: 1999. Contact information: www.ams.org.

The Elements of Style, fourth edition, William Strunk Jr. and E.B. White, Boston et al: Allyn and Bacon, 2000. Contact information: www.abacon.com.

Arthur Plotnik, *The Elements of Editing: A Modern Guide for Editors and Journalists*, New York, NY: Collier Books, 1982. Contact information: www.abacon.com.

Chicago Manual of Style, 14th edition. Chicago and London: University of Chicago Press, 1993. Contact information: www.press.uchicago.edu.

About Writing
William Zinsser, *On Writing Well*, sixth edition. New York, NY: Harper Perennial, 1998. Contact information: www.harpercollins.com.

Robert J. Bonk, PhD, *Medical Writing in Drug Development: A Practical Guide for Pharmaceutical Research*, Haworth Press, 1998. Contact information: www.haworthpressinc.com. Selected by Doody's Journal as one of the best health science books of the year

Articles

"The Science of Science Writing," George D. Gopen and Judith A. Swan, *American Scientist*, Volume 78, November-December 1990.

"Clinical Trials: An Overview," Hardeo Sahai, Anwer Khurshid, and Muhammad I. Ageel, *Applied Clinical Trials*, December 1996.

Medical Dictionaries

Dorland's Illustrated Medical Dictionary, 28th edition. Philadelphia et al.: W.B. Saunders Company, 1994. Contact information: www.harcourthealth.com/WBS.

Stedman's Medical Dictionary, 26th edition. Baltimore, et al: Williams & Wilkins. Contact information: www.lww.com.

Freelance Resources
Books

Robert W. Bly, *Secrets of a Freelance Writer: How to Make $85,000 a Year*, New York, NY: Henry Holt and Company, 1990. Contact information: www.henryholt.com, 888-330-8477.

Marian Faux, Successful Freelancing: *The Complete Guide to Establishing and Running Any Kind of Freelance Business*, New York, NY: St. Martin's Press, 1982. Contact information: www.stmartins.com.

Alexander Kopelman. *National Writers Union Guide to Freelance Rates & Standard Practice.* New York, NY, 1995. Contact info: www.NWU.com, 212-254-0279; NWU@netcom.com.

Articles

"A Marketing Primer for Freelance Medical Writers," Lori De Milto, *AMWA Journal*, Vol. 14, No. 2, Spring 1999.

Appendix C

List of Published Paperback Books Written by Anne Hart

Click on underlined link at http://www.newswriting.net to reach publisher's Web site and browse each book and/or read each book's description. Publisher's Web site also is at http://www.iuniverse.com.

1. <u>How to Open a Business Writing and Publishing Memoirs, Gift Books, or Success Stories for Clients: Make Hand-Crafted Personalized History</u> ISBN: 0-595-38083-2

2. <u>Popular Health & Medical Writing for Magazines: How to Turn Current Research & Trends into Salable Feature Articles</u> ISBN: 0-595-35178-6

3. <u>Writing 45-Minute One-Act Plays, Skits, Monologues, & Animation Scripts for Drama Workshops</u>: Adapting Current Events, Social Issues, Life Stories, News & Histories ISBN: 0-595-34597-2

4. <u>Diet Fads, Careers, & Controversies in Nutrition Journalism</u>: How to Organize Term Papers, News, or Debates ISBN: 0-595-37823-4

5. <u>How to Interpret Family History and Ancestry DNA Test Results for Beginners</u>: The Geography and History of Your Relatives ISBN: 0-595-31684-0

6. <u>Cover Letters, Follow-Ups, and Book Proposals</u>: Samples with Templates

ISBN: 0-595-31663-8

7. <u>Writer's Guide to Book Proposals</u>: Templates, Query Letters, & Free Media Publicity
ISBN: 0-595-31673-5

8. <u>Search Your Middle Eastern and European Genealogy:</u> In the Former Ottoman Empire's Records and Online
ISBN: 0-595-31811-8

9. <u>Ancient and Medieval Teenage Diaries:</u> Writing, Righting, and Riding for Righteousness
ISBN: 0-595-32009-0

10. <u>Is Radical Liberalism or Extreme Conservatism a Character Disorder, Mental Disease, or Publicity Campaign?</u>—A Novel of Intrigue—
ISBN: 0-595-31751-0

11. <u>How to Write Plays, Monologues, and Skits from Life Stories, Social Issues, and Current Events</u>—for all Ages.
ISBN: 0-595-31866-5

12. <u>How to Make Money Organizing Information</u>
ISBN: 0-595-23695-2

13. <u>How To Stop Elderly Abuse</u>: A Prevention Guidebook
ISBN: 0-595-23550-6

14. <u>How to Make Money Teaching Online With Your Camcorder and PC</u>: 25 Practical and Creative How-To Start-Ups To Teach Online

ISBN: 0-595-22123-8

15. <u>A Private Eye Called Mama Africa</u>: What's an Egyptian Jewish Female Psycho-Sleuth Doing Fighting Hate Crimes in California?
ISBN: 0-595-18940-7

16. The Freelance Writer's E-Publishing Guidebook: 25+ E-Publishing Home-based Online Writing Businesses to Start for Freelancers
ISBN: 0-595-18952-0

17. The Courage to Be Jewish and the Wife of an Arab Sheik: What's a Jewish Girl from Brooklyn Doing Living as a Bedouin?
ISBN: 0-595-18790-0

18. A Perfect Mitzvah Gift Book: Time Travel with the Kagan's Kids to 10th Century Kiev, "When Jews Of Eastern Europe Had No Hope Other Than The Grace Of The Almighty, The Coming Of The Meshiach, Or The Arrival Of The Khazars."
ISBN: 0-595-38159-6

19. Predictive Medicine for Rookies: Consumer Watchdogs, Reviews, & Genetics Testing Firms Online
ISBN: 0-595-35146-8

20. Four Astronauts and a Kitten: A Mother and Daughter Astronaut Team, the Teen Twin Sons, and Patches, the Kitten: The Intergalactic Friendship Club
ISBN: 0-595-19202-5

21. The Writer's Bible: Digital and Print Media: Skills, Promotion, and Marketing for Novelists, Playwrights, and Script Writers. Writing Entertainment Content for the New and Print Media.
ISBN: 0-595-19305-6

22. New Afghanistan's TV Anchorwoman: A novel of mystery set in the New Afghanistan
ISBN: 0-595-21557-2

23. Tools for Mystery Writers: Writing Suspense Using Hidden Personality Traits
ISBN: 0-595-21747-8

24. The Khazars Will Rise Again!: Mystery Tales of the Khazars
ISBN: 0-595-21830-X

25. <u>Murder in the Women's Studies Department</u>: A Professor Sleuth Novel of Mystery
ISBN: 0-595-21859-8

26. <u>Make Money With Your Camcorder and PC</u>: 25+ Businesses: Make Money With Your Camcorder and Your Personal Computer by Linking Them.
ISBN: 0-595-21864-4

27. <u>Writing What People Buy</u>: 101+ Projects That Get Results
ISBN: 0-595-21936-5

28. <u>Anne Joan Levine</u>, Private Eye: Internal adventure through first-person mystery writer's diary novels
ISBN: 0-595-21860-1

29. <u>Verbal Intercourse</u>: A Darkly Humorous Novel of Interpersonal Couples and Family Communication
ISBN: 0-595-21946-2

30. <u>The Date Who Unleashed Hell</u>: If You Love Me, Why Do You Humiliate Me?
"The Date" Mystery Fiction
ISBN: 0-595-21982-9

31. <u>Cleopatra's Daughter</u>: Global Intercourse
ISBN: 0-595-22021-5

32. <u>Cyber Snoop Nation</u>: The Adventures Of Littanie Webster, Sixteen-Year-Old Genius Private Eye On Internet Radio
ISBN: 0-595-22033-9

33. <u>Counseling Anarchists</u>: We All Marry Our Mirrors—Someone Who Reflects How We Feel About Ourselves. Folding Inside Ourselves: A Novel of Mystery
ISBN: 0-595-22054-1

34. <u>Sacramento Latina</u>: When the One Universal We Have In Common Divides Us
ISBN: 0-595-22061-4

35. <u>Astronauts and Their Cats</u>: At night, the space station is cat-shadow dark
ISBN: 0-595-22330-3

36. <u>How Two Yellow Labs</u> Saved the Space Program: When Smart Dogs Shape Shift in Space
ISBN: 0-595-23181-0

37. <u>The DNA Detectives</u>: Working Against Time
ISBN: 0-595-25339-3

38. <u>How to Interpret Your DNA Test Results</u> For Family History & Ancestry: Scientists Speak Out on Genealogy Joining Genetics
ISBN: 0-595-26334-8

39. <u>Roman Justice</u>: SPQR: Too Roman To Handle
ISBN: 0-595-27282-7

40. <u>How to Make Money Selling Facts</u>: to Non-Traditional Markets
ISBN: 0-595-27842-6

41. <u>Tracing Your Jewish DNA</u> For Family History & Ancestry: Merging a Mosaic of Communities
ISBN: 0-595-28127-3

42. <u>The Beginner's Guide</u> to Interpreting Ethnic DNA Origins for Family History: How Ashkenazi, Sephardi, Mizrahi & Europeans Are Related to Everyone Else
ISBN: 0-595-28306-3

43. <u>Nutritional Genomics</u>—A Consumer's Guide to How Your Genes and Ancestry Respond to Food: Tailoring What You Eat to Your DNA
ISBN: 0-595-29067-1

44. How to Safely Tailor Your Food, Medicines, & Cosmetics to Your Genes: A Consumer's Guide to Genetic Testing Kits from Ancestry to Nourishment
ISBN: 0-595-29403-0

45. One Day Some Schlemiel Will Marry Me, Pay the Bills, and Hug Me.: Parents & Children Kvetch on Arab & Jewish Intermarriage
ISBN: 0-595-29826-5

46. Find Your Personal Adam And Eve: Make DNA-Driven Genealogy Time Capsules
ISBN: 0-595-30633-0

47. Creative Genealogy Projects: Writing Salable Life Stories
ISBN: 0-595-31305-1

48. Power Dating Games: What's Important to Know About the Person You'll Marry
ISBN: 0-595-19186-X

49. Dramatizing 17th Century Family History of Deacon Stephen Hart & Other Early New England Settlers: How to Write Historical Plays, Skits, Biographies, Novels, Stories, or Monologues from Genealogy Records, Social Issues, & Current Events for All Ages
ISBN: 0-595-34345-7

50. Problem-Solving and Cat Tales for the Holidays: Historical—Time-Travel—Adventure
ISBN: 0-595-32692-7

51. 801 Action Verbs for Communicators: Position Yourself First with Action Verbs for Journalists, Speakers, Educators, Students, Resume-Writers, Editors & Travelers
ISBN: 0-595-31911-4

52. Writing 7-Minute Inspirational Life Experience Vignettes: Create and Link 1,500-Word True Stories
ISBN: 0-595-32237-9

53. Large Print Crossword Puzzles for Memory Enhancement : Neuron-Growing Stimulation for the Age-Wise Brain
ISBN: 0-595-35663-X

54. Tracing Your Baltic, Scandinavian, Eastern European, & Middle Eastern Ancestry Online: Finnish, Swedish, Norwegian, Danish, Icelandic, Estonian, Latvian, Polish, Lithuanian, Greek, Macedonian, Bulgarian, Armenian, Hungarian, Eastern European & Middle Eastern Genealogy (All Faiths)
ISBN: 0-595-35773-3

55. 32 Podcasting & Other Businesses to Open Showing People How to Cut Expenses: Get Higher Quality for Less Money
ISBN: 0-595-36083-1

56. Middle Eastern Honor Killings in the USA: (A Thriller)
ISBN: 0-595-36066-1

57. Infant Gender Selection & Personalized Medicine: Consumer's Guide
ISBN: 0-595-36539-6

58. Writing, Financing, & Producing Documentaries: Creating Salable Reality Video
ISBN: 0-595-36633-3

59. How to Turn Poems, Lyrics, & Folklore into Salable Children's Books: Using Humor or Proverbs
ISBN: 0-595-36735-6

60. Job Coach-Life Coach-Executive Coach-Letter & Resume-Writing Service: Step-by-Step Business Startup Manual Step-by-Step Business Startup Manual
ISBN: 0-595-37100-0

61. Where to Find Your Arab-American or Jewish Genealogy Records: Also: Mediterranean, Assyrian, Iranian, Greek & Armenian
ISBN: 0-595-37325-9

62. Cutting Expenses and Getting More for Less: 41+ Ways to Earn an Income from Opportune Living
ISBN: 0-595-34772-X

63. 35 Video Podcasting Careers & Businesses to Start: Step-by-Step Guide for Home-Grown Broadcasters
ISBN: 0-595-37882-X

64. 1700 Ways to Earn Free Book Publicity: Don't Pay to Market Your Writing
ISBN: 0-595-38553-2

65. How to Start Personal Histories and Genealogy Journalism Businesses: Course Template, Syllabus, Writing and Marketing Guide
ISBN: 0-595-38698-9

66. Social Smarts Strategies That Earn Free Book Publicity: Don't Pay to Market Your Writing
ISBN: 0-595-39221-0

67. Creating Family Newsletters & Time Capsules: How to Publish Multimedia Genealogy Periodicals or Gift Booklets
ISBN: 0-595-39872-3

68. 102 Ways to Apply Career Training in Family History/Genealogy: How to Find a Job, Internship, or Create Your Own Business
ISBN: 0-595-41316-1

69. How to Refresh Your Memory by Writing Salable Memoirs with Laughing Walls: A Pop-Culture Course in Reminiscing for Pay
ISBN: 0-595-41527-X

70. Crack the Employment Personality Testing Code: Includes Sample and Practice Tests for Self-Assessment* Expert Advice on How to Prepare Yourself for Every Kind of Test * Give Them The Answer They Want * Assess Your Score (by Anne Hart with George Sheldon) Career Press, 2007
ISBN: (to be announced on my Web site at http://www.newswriting.net when book becomes available in 2007)

Index

978-0-595-41679-0
0-595-41679-9